4/2/69 $10

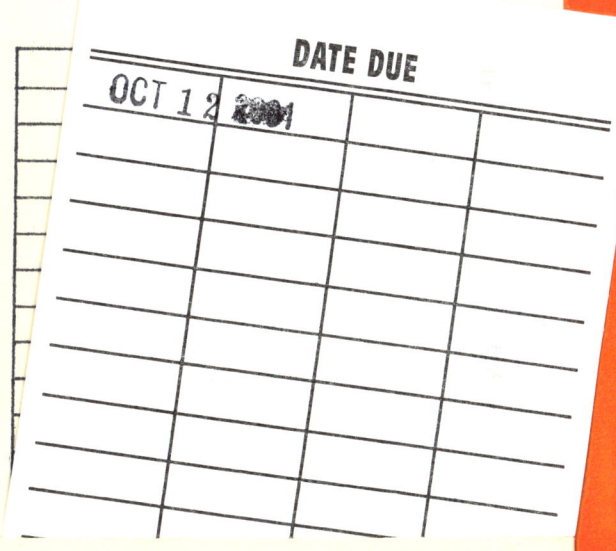

A SINGULAR VIEW
The Art of Seeing With One Eye

For my wife, Lou

A SINGULAR VIEW
The Art of Seeing With One Eye

By Frank B. Brady

with a Foreword by
John W. McTigue, M.D., F.A.C.S.
and illustrations by John Benton Brady

Design by A. Michael Velthaus

Medical Economics Company
Oradell, New Jersey 07649

PUBLISHER'S NOTES:

Frank B. Brady, author of this book, is a resident of Westmoreland Hills, Maryland. He has a broad background in aviation and electronics and is presently employed by the Singer Company's Kearfott Division as a senior staff consultant for technical programs concerned with all-weather landing systems, air navigation, aircraft instrumentation and airport lighting systems.

Thus, in writing this book, Mr. Brady was able to draw both on professional education and his scientific and technical work experience in coping with the problems resulting from loss of vision in one eye. He is also the author or co-author of some two dozen technical papers, articles and reports in various fields of aviation technology.

John W. McTigue, M.D., F.A.C.S., who wrote the Foreword and served as medical consultant for this book, is chief of the department of ophthalmology at the Washington Medical Center in the District of Columbia. His primary professional interests are diseases and surgery involving the cornea. He is the author or co-author of more than 20 professional papers in the specialty of ophthalmology.

John Benton Brady, son of the author, developed the illustrations for this book. He currently is a student at Cornell University in Ithaca, New York.

Copyright © 1972 by Medical Economics Company, Oradell, N.J. 07649. All rights reserved. None of the content of this publication may be reproduced, stored in a retrieval system, or transmitted in any form or by any means (electronic, mechanical, photocopying, recording, or otherwise) without the prior written permission of the publisher.

CONTENTS

Chapter		Page
	FOREWORD	VII
	PREFACE	XII
	ACKNOWLEDGMENTS	XIV
1	UNHAPPY LANDING	1
2	AWKWARD TAKEOFF	3
3	JOLTS OF REALITY	7
4	FLYING HIGH	10
5	HOW ABOUT YOU?	13
6	SEEING IN 3-D	17
7	WHAT'S CHANGED?	21
8	GETTING BACK TO 3-D	31
9	PITFALLS AND BOOBY-TRAPS	40
10	IN THE DRIVER'S SEAT	56
11	THE ACTIVE LIFE	61
12	GIMMICKS AND GADGETS	67
13	KEEPING THE GOOD EYE GOOD	81
14	SEEING TO YOUR LOOKS	89
15	DRIVER AND PILOT LICENSING STANDARDS	95
16	GREAT COMPANY	103

JACKSON COMMUNITY COLLEGE LIBRARY
2111 EMMONS ROAD
JACKSON, MICHIGAN 49201

FOREWORD

By John W. McTigue, M.D., F.A.C.S.*

When Frank Brady told me that he was toying with the idea of writing "a sort of manual for the newly one-eyed," my response was instant and positive. "This is a book that should be written," I told him, "and you are the man to do it."

Frank Brady can speak with the authority of a person who was forced to adjust to the loss of an eye in the very prime of his life. Because of his extensive background in air navigation and in developing ways of landing planes under poor visibility conditions, he was quickly able to understand the problems created by the destruction of so complex an instrument as the human eye.

---

*Dr. McTigue is chief of the department of ophthalmology at the Washington Medical Center in the District of Columbia. He is past president of the District of Columbia Medical Society's section on ophthalmology; past president of the Prevention of Blindness Society, Washington, D.C.; associate medical director of the International Eye Foundation, Washington, D.C., and a member of the board of directors of the Eye Bank Association of America.

And he tackled those problems with an uncanny problem-solving ability.

In no time he was driving a car, flying a plane, courting a girl, plunging into sports with skill and enthusiasm and working as effectively as ever at his highly technical job.

Mr. Brady's remarkable adaptation was made almost entirely without benefit of guidance—because, as he discovered soon after leaving the hospital, no such guidance was available. There are schools and training centers and books aplenty for persons with practically any type of handicap you can name, including those totally without sight. Yet as far as I know, there has never been anything even vaguely resembling this sort of "manual for the newly one-eyed."

A child born with only one good eye, or who loses vision in one eye at a very early age, never faces the kind of adjustment problems that plagued Frank Brady after his accident. A one-eyed child will adapt to his limited vision as naturally as the normal child does to binocular sight. Unconsciously, and unselfconsciously, he'll learn a whole battery of compensating techniques that the child with two good eyes never needs to know—techniques for gauging depth and distance and for enlarging his somewhat restricted field of vision.

The fact that such a child can go on to lead a completely normal life—without any sense of being handicapped—should, I suppose, give hope and reassurance to the person who loses an eye after growing up. Indeed, for him a return to normal living is equally possible. Yet I'm afraid this crumb of comfort isn't sufficient to help him through the often difficult period of adapting to his new situation.

Each year an estimated 50,000 Americans enter the world of the one-eyed—most of them without any advance notice. The loss of an eye is usually sudden and traumatic—by injury or accident—and may plunge its victim into an immediate depression. Reminding him that little Alfie, who was *born* with only one eye, has just graduated at the top of his class isn't going to cheer an adult victim very much.

Nor will it help him cope with the immediate problems and vexations he'll encounter in everyday activities—all the errors of visual judgment that will make him feel anxious, clumsy, foolish. The ophthalmologist may tell him he's going to "get along just great," but rarely does a busy physician have time to sit down with such a patient and explain precisely *how* to "get along just great." Even if he did, he could never have that special understanding of the patient's problems that can only come from experiencing them.

This book fills that gap admirably. The author starts out with a vivid though understated description of his accident and his feelings when he learned that his damaged eye would have to be removed. He recounts the tribulations and failures in his early efforts to get back to his old way of life with his new restriction. He tells us how he mastered each of his problems in turn.

There follows a remarkably condensed and simplified basic course on how the human eyes function, with particular reference to depth perception and visual field. We learn exactly what's lost and what's necessary for an intelligent adaptation to living with monocular vision.

I particularly like the chapters that follow—the nuts-and-bolts of the book. Here Mr. Brady explains his precise techniques for shaking a hand without missing, for stepping off a curb without stumbling, for guiding a car through a narrow lane or a thread through a needle's eye. He makes the obstacles and pitfalls appear much less challenging as he leads us on through the world of gadgetry— glasses, magnifiers, rangefinders, offset gunsights and other ingenious devices to improve performance of specific tasks.

Frank Brady's observations on lighting, a field that cries out for more research, may prove to be a pioneering contribution.

The next chapter—the one he discussed most with me—tells the newly one-eyed how to care for and make the most of the precious eye that's left.

This is followed by a trove of useful information on licensing requirements for car drivers and plane pilots. The book ends with a reminder that loss of an eye late in life didn't cramp the style or detract from the achievements of some world-famous people working in a variety of fields.

While this manual is addressed primarily to the newly one-eyed, I hope that it will reach the much larger audience it deserves. It should make almost equally good reading for those who have long ago adapted to what Mr. Brady refers to, not as a handicap, but as "this inconvenience," or "this damned nuisance."

I think this book will also interest anyone who is curious about the workings of one of nature's most fabulous creations—the human eye. And it will certainly captivate every person who enjoys reading about man's amazing capacity for adaptation.

PREFACE

A man's eyes are his closest bond to his environment, and any threat to his vision is certain to produce massive anxieties. Even the loss of *one* eye can be a matter of enormous concern to an active individual in love with living. Will he ever again, he wonders, be able to work, to drive, to fly, to hunt, to win a mate?

I went through all these anxieties when I lost my own good right eye, but I suppose I tended to feel that my reactions were exceptional. It really wasn't until friends began to call on me to help reassure others who had recently lost an eye that I began to understand how deep can be the psychological trauma inflicted by loss of an eye.

These sessions also brought home to me the fact that there is very little guidance for the newly one-eyed during the long, awkward and sometimes dangerous period of adaptation. My own experiences while getting used to monocular vision had caused me to develop techniques I now was able to pass on to newcomers—practical suggestions that could help them over the curbs and stairways and other stumbling blocks on the road to normalcy.

Eventually, I began to wonder if these techniques might not be equally helpful to a much larger number of people if I could properly communicate them. Slowly the idea formed of putting together a sort of manual on how to see with one eye. And so this book was born.

I had to learn most of the techniques I've explained here the hard way, as I suspect most other victims of this inconvenience have been forced to do. But it's my hope that this book will spare others some of the bumps and bruises I acquired trying to figure things out on my own.

—FRANK B. BRADY

ACKNOWLEDGMENTS

One of the most pleasant surprises connected with the preparation of this book has been the enthusiastic response to almost any request for assistance. I couldn't possibly acknowledge all the help I've received from individuals and organizations, but I do want to mention a few that have been especially generous in their response. These include:

The American Medical Association's Committee on Medical Aspects of Automotive Safety.

The Federal Aviation Administration, Office of the Flight Surgeon.

The American Association of Motor Vehicle Administrators.

The American Optical Corporation.

The Guild of Prescription Opticians of America.

Mr. Joseph Murphy, editor and publisher of *Air Transport Magazine*, who helped me find a publisher.

My acknowledgments wouldn't be complete without a word of appreciation for Dr. Wendell Hughes, the eminent New York ophthalmologist whose skill and patience in the performance of five operations over a two-year period succeeded in rebuilding my battered features.

And finally, a heartfelt thank-you to Dr. John W. McTigue, the distinguished ophthalmologist in Washington, D.C., without whose encouragement, prodding and generous assistance this book might never have got beyond the procrastination stage.

1

UNHAPPY LANDING

I have no memory of being hit. I recall only a dazed awareness that something was wrong, very wrong ... that Charles Macatee was swinging our plane into position for a landing ... asking the tower for runway lights ... calling for an ambulance to meet the plane.

Then Tom Wright, the third man aboard, was helping me out of the cockpit, where I had been flying copilot, and onto a couch so that he could take my place and assist in the landing.

Interminable minutes later (less than three, actually) I was being lifted into the ambulance for a trip that clanged through an eternity of night. Exactly seven minutes after the accident I was getting skilled emergency treatment in an Air Force hospital.

Our plane, a research DC-3, had been on the last leg of a flight from Chicago via Washington that April evening. We'd been skimming over Long Island after sunset and were preparing to land at Grumman Field, our home base, when the craft was struck. Captain Macatee (who later was to pilot the first scheduled jetliner across the American continent) had no idea what had hit us until after landing, when a five-pound mallard duck was found in the cockpit, battered but intact.

The big bird, one of a migrating pair that had collided with us, had crashed through the windshield and struck me full in the face, bouncing my head against the aluminum bulkhead behind me. A large dent in the heavy metal testified to the force of that blow. Later, when I had a chance to examine it, I realized that the bulkhead had actually saved my neck from snapping under the impact—that I was lucky to be alive.

As a result of my work on aviation safety, I had recently taken a keen interest in tests designed to strengthen cockpit windshields against just such bird strikes—which had already been fatal to a number of fliers. The method was to fire a newly killed chicken encased in a paper bag from a pneumatic cannon at various types of windshield mock-ups. The technique is still in use today, except that the chickens are now fired at velocities as high as 700 miles an hour. Thanks to such testing, the modern cockpit windshield is an inch-thick marvel of strength, with heated laminations to prevent its becoming brittle at high-altitude temperatures.

By a wry twist of fate, stronger windshields had been ordered installed on all DC-3s. Ours arrived shortly after the accident.

2

AWKWARD TAKEOFF

It was several days before the doctors decided I was strong enough to hear the bad news: My right eye was damaged beyond repair. It would have to be removed without delay, they told me, to prevent a sympathetic reaction from developing in the remaining eye.

The verdict didn't really surprise me, even though the damaged eye had been kept under wraps all this time. And there was really no point in brooding about it. I began instead to develop an overwhelming curiosity about the future. Would my world be changed when viewed through a single eye? Would my activities be restricted? Would I ever drive a car again? Fly a plane? Play golf or even just cross a street with a reasonable expectation of reaching the other side alive?

In the course of my life I'd met quite a few people who had lost the vision of one eye. Now I spent long hours in my hospital bed anxiously trying to recall all the details I'd learned about them so I could apply this knowledge to my own circumstances.

There was Bob, for instance, who wore a patch on one eye and delighted in driving his car at 90 miles an hour on winding rural roads, scattering alarm throughout the countryside. I had no desire to duplicate Bob's madness, but at least it was heartening to think that the loss of half his vision had restrained him no more than the laws of the land.

On the other hand, I knew that Bob had lost his eye at a very early age, and I wondered if this might not be the key to his amazing adaptation. Could I, already past 30, hope to win back enough of my old skills to continue the life I'd been leading—to say nothing of acquiring some necessary new skills?

My thoughts turned, more hopefully, to another acquaintance—one who had lost an eye when he was already a grown man. Cliff, a coworker of mine in an engineering lab, was respected by all of us for his impeccable craftsmanship. He had often discussed with me some of the techniques he used to gauge distances and manipulate instruments—techniques that were presently to serve me well.

Then there was the great Wiley Post, one of my boyhood heroes. With only the relatively crude instruments of the period, Post had twice circled the globe by air with only one good eye to guide him. Pondering his long solo flights and his many landings under the most difficult conditions helped to convince me that the loss of one eye need not *necessarily* be a severe handicap for the rest of my life.

So my mind drove on, searching out reasons for optimism and answers to doubts. But the trip wasn't all upbeat. A hospital environment has a way of magnifying fears and misgivings, especially at night, and there were times when I felt agonizingly sure that neither my personal nor my professional life would ever be the same again.

On the day set for my departure, a pleasant young man came into my room and introduced himself as Dr. Drake.

"How're you doing?" he asked.

"Just fine," I answered truthfully. The prospect of getting back into action at last had buoyed my spirits.

Dr. Drake sat down and began what seemed to be a very casual, amiable and innocent conversation. But little by little his questions became more penetrating, dwelling especially on my general outlook about life. He wanted to know whether it had changed since the accident.

It was only near the end of the interview that I began to realize I was on the receiving end of a very skillful psychiatric examination. Dr. Drake's purpose, obviously, was to find out whether the loss of an eye and the battering of the whole right half of my face had thrown me into a depression.

The effect of the interview, however, was to raise

my mood almost to the point of elation. I began to feel a bit like a boy in the story who asked the doctor, after surgery on his hands, "Will I be able to play piano now?"

"Definitely," said the doctor.

"Wow!" screamed the boy. "That's great! I could never do *that* before."

Apparently I emerged from the interview with passing marks, for when Dr. Drake rose to go he wished me good-bye and good luck.

I reached to grasp his outstretched hand—and missed by a mile!

JOLTS OF REALITY

It didn't take me too long to master the art of handshaking, but the real world that was waiting to wake me up from my hospital daydreams had many more rude jolts in store for me.

Outside the hospital I stepped off the sidewalk to hail a cab. Underestimating the height of the curb, I jolted forward and nearly ended up under the taxi's wheels.

At a party in my honor I volunteered to mix a martini for a thirsty young woman. I mixed it perfectly. Then, when she held up her glass to receive it, I poured it on the floor.

My "grand entrance" at another party became a spectacle. I descended the stairs, raised my hands in greeting to the guests, stepped into the living room, and fell forward in amazement. The last step had disguised itself as part of the living room floor.

My first try at table tennis was a disaster that stirred my friends to a pitying quietness.

It seemed everybody in the world had suddenly decided to move in on my right (sightless) side, and I was in a constant state of collision with them. A restaurant waitress serving hot soup on my right came up just as my hands were describing the size of a fish I'd once caught. I caught the plate this time, and a painful burn that lingered on my right arm for several days—evidence of a newborn clumsiness.

For some time I was to live in a world of clumsiness and embarrassments, much of which I could have been spared if only someone had given me the explanations and helpful tips that appear in the following chapters.

It was perhaps with justifiable trepidation that at the urging of friends I got behind the wheel of a car less than two days after leaving the hospital. I tried to cling to the right lane, but there were the parked cars, the double-parked cars and the intersections, where terrors seemed to spill in from all directions—but particularly from the right.

I had to swivel my head in much wider arcs, much faster and much more frequently than I ever had before in the driver's seat, and it needed a more finely honed sense of alertness to cope with each new danger. I was pathetically grateful for the "copilot" on my right during that first nightmarish ride through town.

Out on the open highway, however, things went smoother and some of my old sense of ease at the wheel returned. I did become aware, however, of a tendency to overrun the car ahead. But I quickly learned to lag a little farther than usual behind vehicles and soon began to understand why my old friend Bob had no qualms about going 90 miles an hour once his path was clear of traffic.

It was while driving at slow speeds, threading my way between other cars on the city streets or backing into a parking space that I experienced the most serious difficulty in judging distances. Nevertheless, I ended that first drive with certainty that this was one activity I wouldn't have to give up, for at no time had I felt that I was driving in an unsafe manner. Any loss of visual perception was more than offset by the enforced—and often excruciating—increase in alertness.

4

FLYING HIGH

That same superalertness sustained me as I tested myself in a variety of skills for which I had a well established know-how—but also a recently acquired uneasiness about my do-how. For it was back in my boyhood that I had begun acquiring the assortment of knacks and knowledges that later guided my choice of a career.

At 16 I was a glider buff, obtaining my pilot's license in a craft that school chums and I had built and taught ourselves to fly. Soon after that I became fascinated by ham radio, building and operating amateur stations. And as I grew up I was drawn almost painlessly into the field of radio engineering. My old interest in flying, however, caused me to turn to aviation electronics, where I found a new specialty—the development of instrument approach and landing systems.

World War II created a demand for men with this type of background, and as a young civilian engineer I was soon in charge of a sizable instrument landing program for Allied Forces in Europe. After the war I joined the civil aviation industry to help the airlines adapt the new air traffic control and instrument landing systems to peacetime use. It was in this capacity that I was directing a flight research program on the night of the accident.

Though my main interest had always been my work, I don't think I was backward in social or outdoor activities. Swimming and sailing were my favorite sports, augmented by a bit of tennis and golf. Now each of these old activities presented new challenges as I cautiously experimented and, problem by problem, worked out ways of coping.

Shortly after the accident I was back at my job and having no difficulty filling it. The flight research program had been dropped, so I was no longer required to fly. I flew anyway—partly to find out how I'd do at it and partly because it's in my blood. In many ways I found it easier than driving, and I had no trouble with the distance judgments required for landing and other maneuvers.

Even today, with increased air traffic making it imperative for a pilot to keep a sharp lookout in the sky, I find that the superalertness I've trained into myself easily compensates for the loss of side vision. In fact, I would go so far as to say that there is a *net gain* in safety.

Perhaps my most demanding post-accident project was the building of a ship model to exacting standards. It's true that threading all those tiny deadeyes, setting up the rigging at a scale of one-eighth inch to the foot and doing all the other fine detailed work wasn't easy; the point is that it was possible—and that it was done with no loss of quality in the workmanship.

All in all, my adaptation was well along at the end of a year. By the end of two years I was totally at ease in all normal activities, even though I was, for cosmetic reasons, still undergoing plastic surgery. Some jobs took a little extra time and effort, and many situations called for the hyperawareness I've already mentioned. But if I sometimes regarded my new condition as a damned nuisance, I never considered it a handicap—in my career, in my hobbies, or in my personal life.

It was toward the end of this rehabilitation period that, through a chance meeting, my personal life took a highly affirmative turn and the success of my adaptation was proved by the fact that for months I made weekly trips from Washington up through Maryland and Pennsylvania, driving seven hours at a stretch— and mostly at night—to woo the future Mrs. Brady.

5

HOW ABOUT YOU?

So much for my story. Now what about yours? If you're reading this book, the chances are that you have just lost, or are in the process of losing, the full use of one eye. In the months ahead—those months that now occupy all your thoughts—will you fare as well as I did? Better? Worse? Let's take a look at some of the factors that may help or hinder you on the road back.

Every person is right-eyed or left-eyed, just as he is right-handed or left-handed, depending on which half of the brain is dominant. The right hand, foot and eye are controlled by the left hemisphere of the brain, which in most persons is dominant. Obviously, the loss of your right hand, if that's the favored one, would call for a far longer and more difficult readjustment than loss of the left; it would entail a massive reeducation of the brain.

To a lesser extent the same holds true of the eyes. If your brain is accustomed to receiving messages and making decisions on the basis of information received from your right eye, and that's the one you lose, the road back's going to be a bit more arduous for you. In my own case it was the right, or favored, eye that was removed, so it was a minus factor for me.

While eye dominance is perhaps the single most important factor in the prognosis, there are many others that play a part. One of these is acuity of vision. If the surviving eye has good vision (as in my case), it can more readily take over the functions of its lost mate, even though that mate may have been the favored one. But if the surviving eye has poor vision and is also the secondary eye, then it's going to take more time and effort to adjust.

Age, of course, is another important factor (the younger you are, the better). So is the gradualness or the suddenness of the loss. If the deterioration of one eye goes on over a long period of time, the good eye has a chance to accustom itself slowly to the increased workload and make an orderly transition. That is, provided the deterioration doesn't cause bothersome symptoms that could retard your adaptation.

Then, of course, much depends on how far you want or need to carry your adaptation. Some occupations (such as mine) and some hobbies (such as mine) call for more accurate depth perception than is normally required. Achieving this requires a longer and more determined effort than average, too.

Of extreme importance is each individual's

psychological reaction to the loss of an eye. And here the difference can be striking, ranging all the way from "What's the use of living?" to "I hardly notice the difference."

One night, while I was still in the early stages of my own recovery, I got an urgent call from a friend asking whether I would please talk with his 18-year-old nephew, who had recently lost an eye as the result of an auto accident. Fred, he said, had come home from the hospital in such a severe state of depression that his family was greatly concerned about what he might do. I readily agreed to visit him as it seemed to me that such a visit might also be helpful to me.

It turned out that Fred and I had a lot more in common than the loss of an eye. During our conversation I learned that he was a glider enthusiast, and immediately I was able to talk his language. As soon as we got on that subject he told me the cause of his despair, which, very simply, was the certainty that he would never again fly a glider.

I was able to assure him from my own experience that he was completely mistaken. I told him about some of the tricks I'd learned to compensate for my loss of vision while flying. At last he was convinced, and his mood quickly changed from one of self-destruction to eagerness to get on with his recovery.

But not all psychological reactions to the loss of

an eye are so simple. I've known victims who took it as a punishment for God knows what unspeakable sins they'd committed in their imagination. Others feel they must *over*compensate for the loss by learning to do *more* than they could when they had normal vision. The miseries and frustrations that can come from such reactions sometimes call for prolonged psychiatric help.

On the other hand, some people of great character and determination actually succeed in overcompensating—like Sammy Davis, Jr. When this great entertainer had the top rung practically in his grasp in 1954, his left eye was damaged beyond repair in a car crash. While recuperating he vowed: "When I come back there can be no 'He's almost as good as he ever was.' I've got to be better."

And within four months he was back, this time right at the top of his profession. Nothing sick about that!

6

SEEING IN 3-D

If you've enjoyed fairly normal vision since birth, it may never have occurred to you that much of what we call "seeing" is a learned skill. We tend to take it for granted that any creature born with eyes can "see." But show a dog a photograph of his beloved master, and he'll display no sign of recognition whatever. It takes an educated brain to translate variations in color and shape on a piece of paper into the likeness of a human being.

I once witnessed the reaction of a small boy who was watching his father's plane take off from a private airfield. As the small plane soared away into the blue, the child began to scream.

"Daddy will be back soon," his mother reassured him. But that wasn't what was bothering the boy.

"Look!" he screamed even louder, pointing to the tiny speck in the sky, "Daddy's getting *small!*"

The youngster was only confirming what scientific studies have found—that the gift of sight doesn't necessarily endow a person with "perception," or the ability to grasp the meaning of what he sees. Persons who have been blind from birth, and then suddenly have eyesight conferred on them by surgery or some other technique, have a whole new language to learn. It takes them some time, for instance, before they can interpret perspective in a picture—just as it must have taken the little boy some time to learn to relate small size to distance.

In the same way, partial loss of the vision you've learned and have used all your life entails a whole new learning experience. But there's a tendency among persons who've always had normal vision to make the transition from two eyes to one by letting nature take its course. This unorganized approach will eventually get you there, but you can speed it up and smooth it out significantly by doing a bit of homework. The first thing you need to understand is the nature of the change that has taken place. What is it, exactly, that you have lost? And what is it that you have left?

The human eye is certainly one of nature's most amazing creations. Just as man stands at the top of the evolutionary ladder, vision is the most highly developed of the senses. Each eyeball is in reality a superbly crafted sub-subminiature camera. When both these cameras are in good working order, their owner need only flip open his lids to obtain a continuous view of the world in glorious 3-D living color.

Most owners use their cameras for fixed viewing about 90 per cent of the time. During the re-

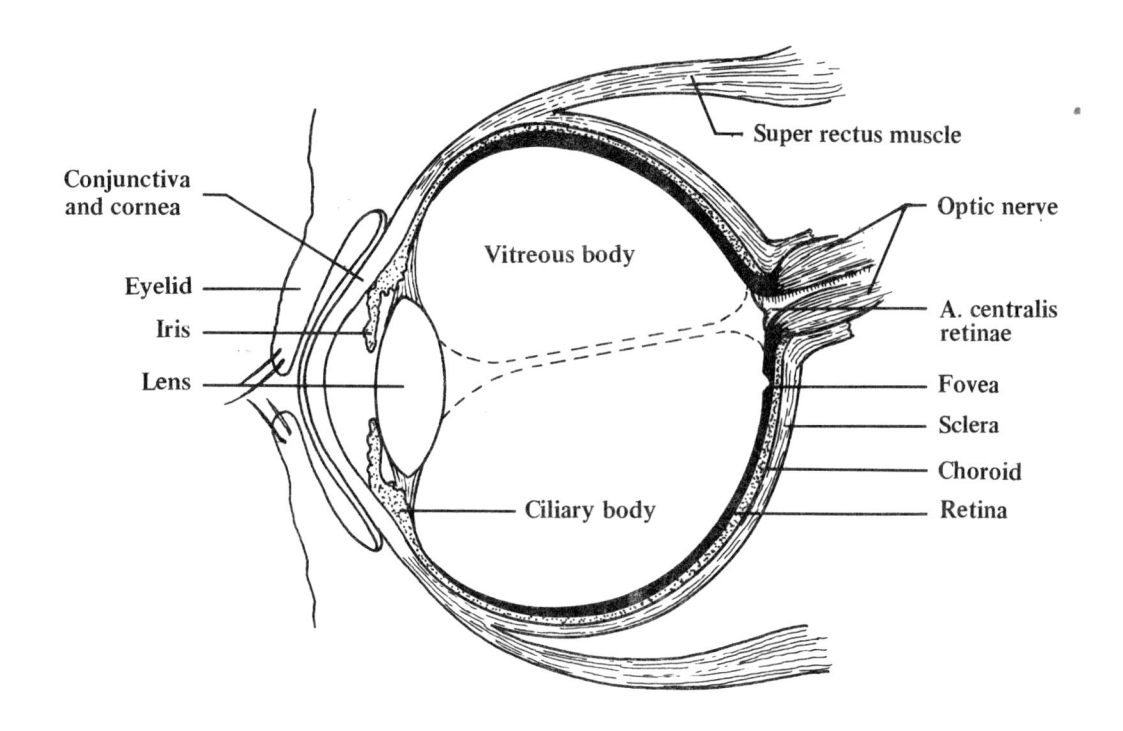

Sectional diagram of the human eye.

maining 10 per cent, the cameras swivel back and forth, up and down, in a series of rapid movements, scanning various parts of the scene at the rate of two or three "takes" per second.

Any part of the big scene that commands the owner's attention, whether it be the top of a mountain or the eye of a needle, first enters the eye through the cornea. This tough, transparent outer shell of the eyeball serves two purposes: (1) it protects the delicate mechanisms from injury, and (2) its front surface bends the rays of light passing through it to form the image on the retina. The lens, by changing shape, provides the change in focus required for viewing near and far objects.

The retina, of course, corresponds to the sensitive film of the movie camera. And just as the images can be stored on film, so the brain can preserve them in its memory file.

The tiny section of the retina called the fovea has special properties. It can exercise the finest color discrimination and record the most delicate images with great clarity. It is the jeweler's loupe for investigating the point of interest.

For the benefit of shutterbugs, here are some technical specifications of the human eye:

It has an f3.5 lens with focal length of approximately 1 inch. It provides automatic focusing from 4 inches to infinity. Each eye's lateral field of view would be a full 180 degrees, except for the bridge of the nose, which restricts it to about 160 degrees. The iris automatically adjusts the pupil opening by a factor of 16 to 1 to accommodate extremely wide variations in light levels. The eye sees in such detail that it can resolve about 10 line pairs per millimeter at normal reading distance.

It's true that a hawk can see better than a man at great distances, and that a cat can see better in the dark. But for man's all-around viewing purposes, there is certainly nothing better than a human eye.

Except, perhaps, two of them.

7

WHAT'S CHANGED?

What happens, physiologically, when you lose one of those two optical marvels with which you've been viewing the world? You know, as soon as you step back out into that world, that *something* has happened, because it has suddenly been transformed into a china closet. Your adaptation to this new and uncomfortable environment can be speeded by an elementary understanding of what's taken place *inside* of you.

Three things have happened:
1. Your horizontal field of vision has narrowed.
2. Your depth perception has been impaired.
3. Your whole visual system, including brain and motor functions, is in disarray and needs reprogramming.

Other, minor, effects will be touched on later. But first let's consider these three important ones.

FIELD OF VISION

You've literally lost out by a nose here. As we've remarked in the last chapter, each eye has a lens capable of taking in everything on the horizon within 180 degrees, or a full half-circle. But that bony prominence in the middle of your face cuts off anywhere from 20 to 40 degrees of that view, depending, naturally, on its size and shape.

This was no problem, of course, so long as you had a good eye on the other side of your nose. Each eye was then able to stand sentinel over that area its mate couldn't cover.

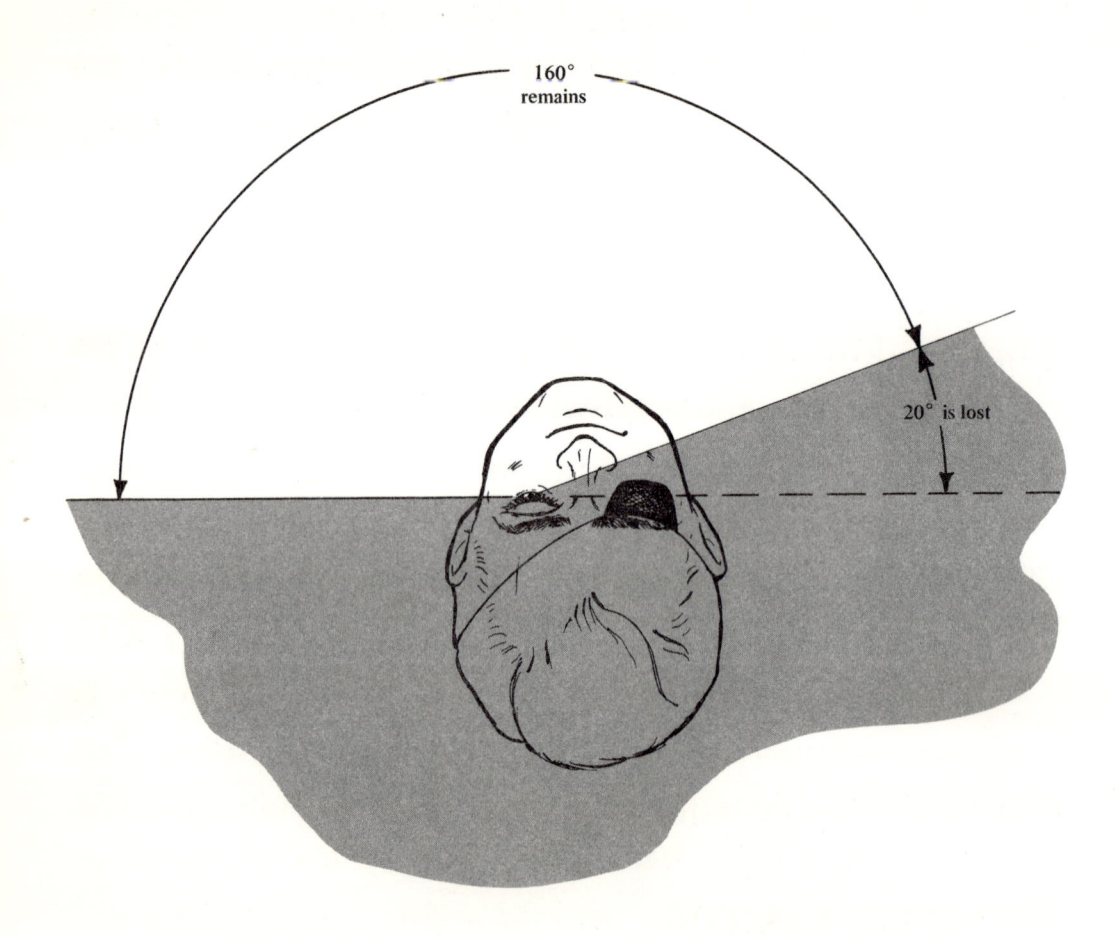

Depending on nose size, the horizontal field for one eye will encompass up to 160°, compared with a 180° field for normal, two-eyed vision.

With one eye gone, the total field of view once covered by both your eyes has been reduced by 10 to 20 per cent, and all of that reduction is on the side of the missing or nonfunctioning eye. That side, as you've already surmised from reading about my difficulties, is where the danger lurks—especially during the early stages of recovery.

Actually there's more nuisance than danger, once you've made adjustments to your new limitation. If the loss of lateral vision seems enormous to you—as it usually does at first—keep in mind that it's really less than many persons with two good eyes inflict on themselves voluntarily by wearing heavy-rimmed glasses.

Your *vertical* field of vision, which totals around 130 degrees, won't be affected.

DEPTH PERCEPTION

The mechanisms by which we judge the size of an object and its distance from us are much more complex than most people realize. In part this is because psychological factors often have an important influence on such judgments. If, for example, you lay a quarter and a metal washer the same size on a table and ask an underprivileged child to tell you which is larger, the odds are heavy that he'll choose the quarter.

But depth perception also involves several pretty

sophisticated *physiological* operations, known in medical terminology as retinal disparity, convergence and accommodation.

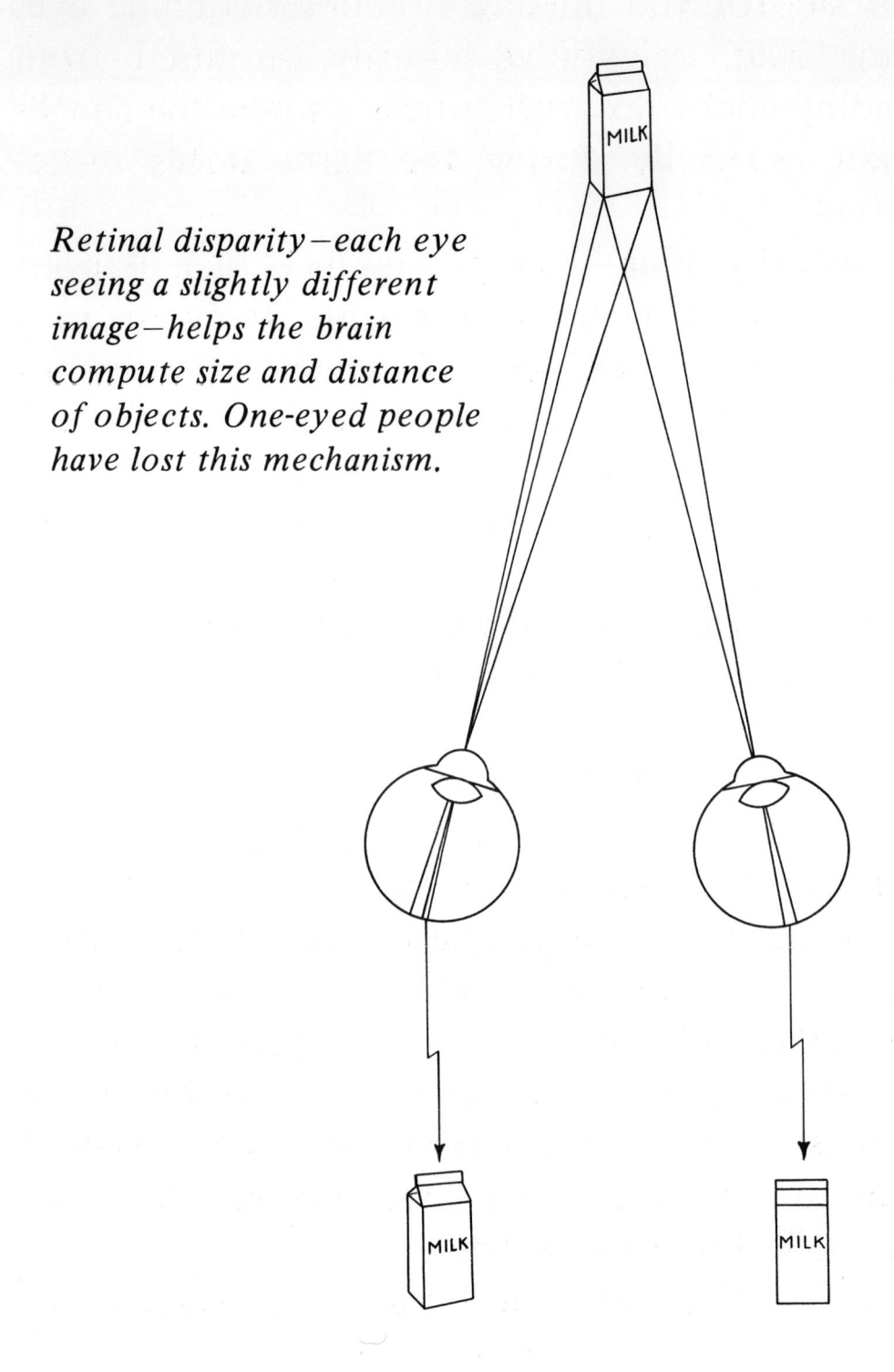

Retinal disparity—each eye seeing a slightly different image—helps the brain compute size and distance of objects. One-eyed people have lost this mechanism.

Retinal disparity is the most obvious and widely known of these mechanisms. It depends on an object being viewed with two eyes separated by several inches so that each is looking at the same target from a slightly different location at the same moment. One eye sees a little way around to the right of the object, and the other eye a little way around to the left. The result: Two slightly different images are produced on the two retinas. Before these images are merged into one clear picture, the brain examines the differences and uses them to make a swift computation of the object's size and distance.

Since the differences diminish rapidly with distance, this mechanism is of little use for remote objects, and no use at all for the person who no longer has two good eyes.

Convergence has to do with the merging of the two images produced on the retinas by the mechanism just described. The effort by the eyes to bring the two images into exact correspondence produces a strain, or torsion, on each eye, and the experienced brain knows how to translate this into a measure of distance. The closer the object, the greater (and more measurable) the torsion. And if you've ever looked crosseyed at a pencil held vertically in front of your nose, you've experienced this strain at its extreme.

Like the mechanism of retinal disparity, convergence is useful only at relatively small distances (25 feet or less), and only to people with binocular vision.

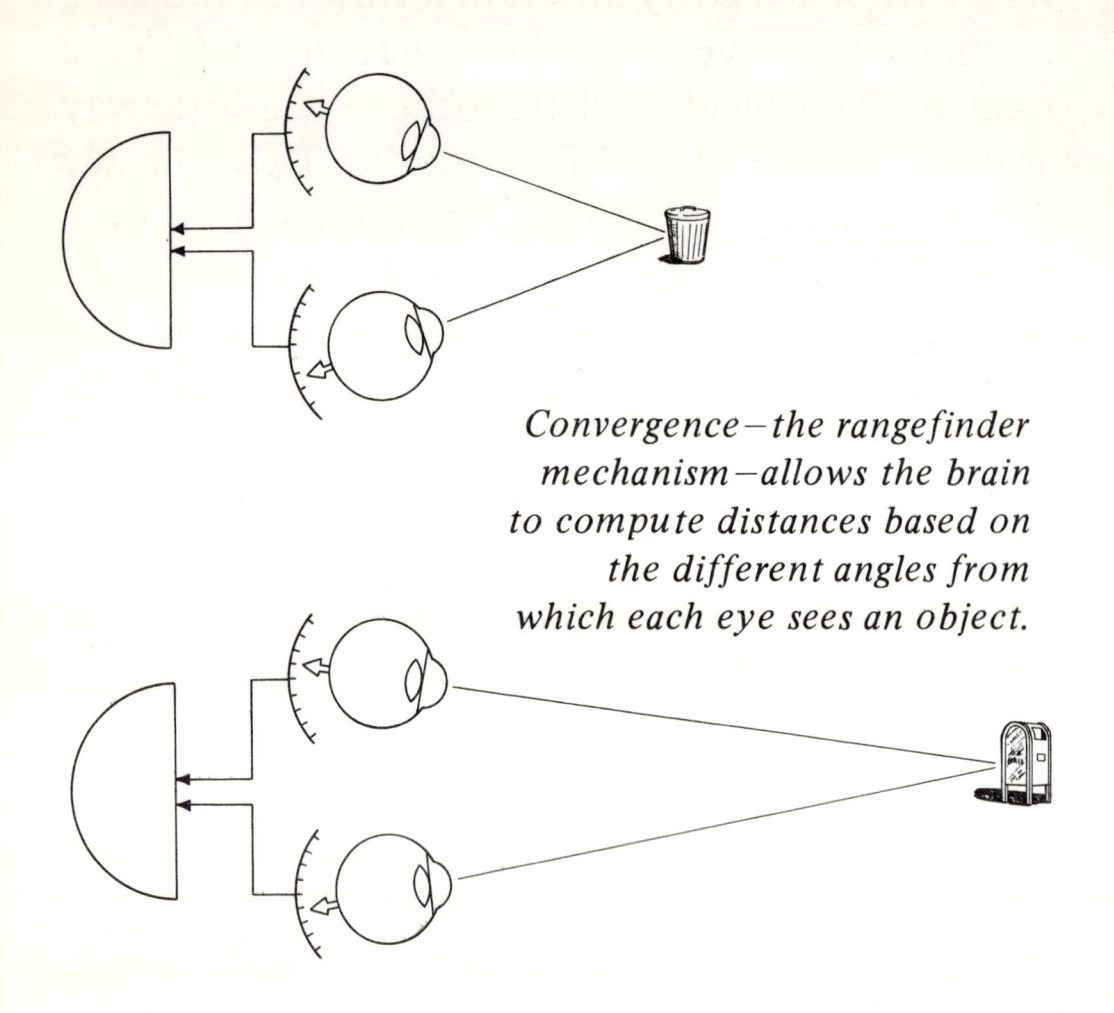

Convergence—the rangefinder mechanism—allows the brain to compute distances based on the different angles from which each eye sees an object.

Accommodation is a term for the automatic adjustment each eye makes to bring an object into focus (as distinct from adjustment, already described, which is then made to merge the two images). This is accomplished by changing the curvature of the lens and the muscular effort

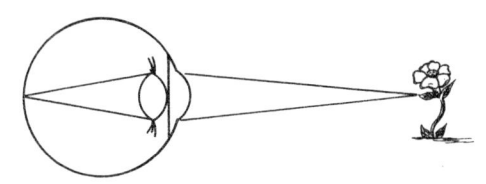

Accommodation—the change in curvature of the lens to bring objects into focus—is immediately interpreted by the brain as a measure of distance.

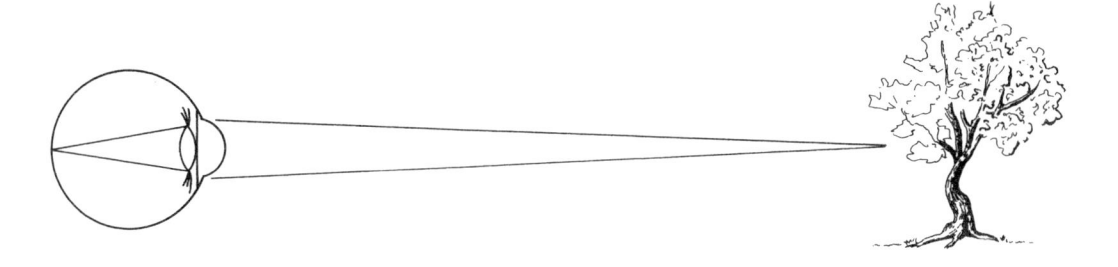

required to do so is immediately registered on the brain as a measure of distance.

Accommodation is only effective for judging distances up to about 6 feet; thus it's likely to be the least useful of the three mechanisms. But it's the only one left to you when you've lost an eye, so cultivate it for what it's worth. You'll soon learn, however, that there's greater gain in developing new techniques to compensate for the loss of retinal disparity and convergence.

Bear in mind, too, that compensation is necessary only up to a point. R. L. Gregory of Cambridge University's psychology department notes in his book *Eye and Brain* that *all* sighted persons "are effectively one-eyed for distances greater than 20 feet."

THE VISUAL SYSTEM

The relationship between your eyes, your brain and your body is something that's been developing since the day you were born. Seeing is only a part of the visual process, which calls for all elements of the system to respond to each other with amazing swiftness and sensitivity.

Even as you read this book, your brain, receiving a signal from your eye, consults its own vast memory bank in order to make a judgment about it—to act, that is, on the basis of experience. It then sends out its commands via the nervous system to activate the body's motor systems. "Turn the page," says your brain, and your fingers obey.

What happens when your brain receives an impaired or different visual message—one for which it has no precedent in its memory bank? To understand how the visual system can be disorganized, let's picture a batter who is about to swing at a pitched ball.

He's trained himself to judge the speed and path of the ball by any or all of the three physiological depth perception processes we've just talked about. A fourth factor he sometimes brings into his computations is the angle at which the ball is approaching the plate. The angle changes as the ball nears, and the brain has the ability to convert the information on the degree of change into a prediction as to where and when the ball will cross the plate. Having digested all available information, the brain at the proper instant sends out a command to the proper muscles to swing the bat. Then, if all goes well, the ball and bat connect solidly at exactly the right juncture in time and place.

But suppose we ask this batter to close one eye and repeat the performance. Only one of the three built-in depth perception techniques—accommodation—is now available to him. And as we know, it won't do him any good until the ball is practically on top of him. So he's forced to rely very heavily on information derived from the angle of the ball's approach.

But his techniques for observing the angle have not really been sharpened (as they would be if this had always been his sole criterion). His brain's file on the subject of baseball angles is still sparse. In short, it's a good bet that he's going to miss the ball.

Even if he has been a highly skilled ballplayer, a significant part of his skill will be lost in the transition from dual to single vision. If instead of just closing one eye experimentally, our batter had actually lost the use of that eye permanently, he would have to develop a whole new set of skills. He would have to supply his brain with a whole new complex of signals and experiences to store up for future reference. And if he was a professional, he may never regain the level of skill he had before.

Most amateurs in the same situation, however, should certainly be able to get back enough skill to enjoy the game. And many may find, as I so often did, that a slight loss in ability can be more than made up by an increase in effort and attention. In fact, in many less critical sports than baseball there's no reason why the loss of an eye should be any problem at all.

8

GETTING BACK TO 3-D

Have you ever seen a photographer cover one eye to study a scene before he films it? What he's trying to do, of course, is to view the picture in two dimensions, the way his one-eyed camera will view it.

And that's somewhat the way you'd view the world from now on, if you took the loss of one eye lying down—or sitting still. Sitting in your room with your head motionless, you no longer see a little to the right and a little to the left of every object to give it roundness and depth. Your eyes no longer strain to bring two slightly different images into correspondence on your retinas. Thus deprived of the two most important physiological means of depth perception—retinal disparity and convergence—what you see is a rather flattened-out scene, much like an ordinary photograph.

Now tilt your head back so that your eye moves up a couple of inches. Something happens. Everything in the room shifts position a little. The edge of the chair in front of you seems to go down a trifle, the television console behind it to come up a trifle, so that you now see a bit more of the TV screen. Your brain at once translates the degree of shift into an estimate of the distance between the TV set and the chair, and for an instant you are able to see your surroundings in three dimensions again.

Perhaps your brain's estimate was off by a hair or a hand. No matter. With practice you're going to become quite accurate at this kind of estimating. In fact, it's going to become a way of life with you.

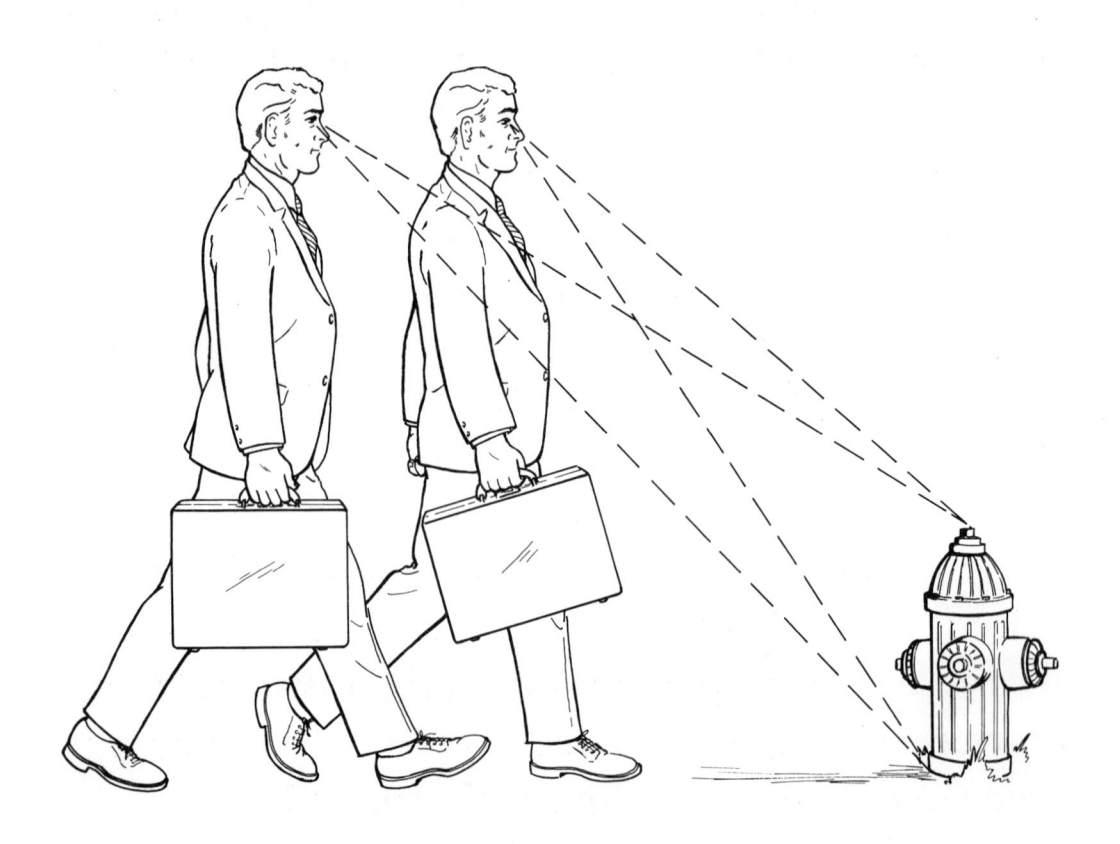

Relative motion—the varying angles and the apparent change in size of objects as you move toward or away from them—will be your primary technique in regaining depth perception.

What has happened? You have created and used the phenomenon of *relative motion*, the same technique used by our hypothetical batter in the last chapter, when he swung at the ball with one eye closed.

Relative motion is one of the two most important methods by which you're going to win your way back into a three-dimensional world and a normal life. The other method is learning to pick up the subtle clues to depth and distance that painters call perspective. Both of these methods are going to be part of your daily living from here on, so let's take a look at each in turn.

RELATIVE MOTION

All of us use this technique constantly as an adjunct to other methods of depth perception—frequently without being aware that we're doing so. For the one-eyed person, a grasp of the principles involved is an important short-cut to full adaptation.

One final reference to our batting friend out there on the field. He was able to use the principle of relative motion because he was standing *to one side* of the plate at which the ball was aimed. Consequently the ball sped toward him at an angle, which kept changing as it approached. Without this angle, his brain would have had little to work on in computing his swing.

Now let's leave the baseball field and move to a tennis court. Here we'll ask you to imagine yourself behind the net with a hard ball coming directly toward you. As it approaches, there's no change in the angle of its path—just an apparent increase in its size, which is not enough information for your brain to accurately compute your swing at it.

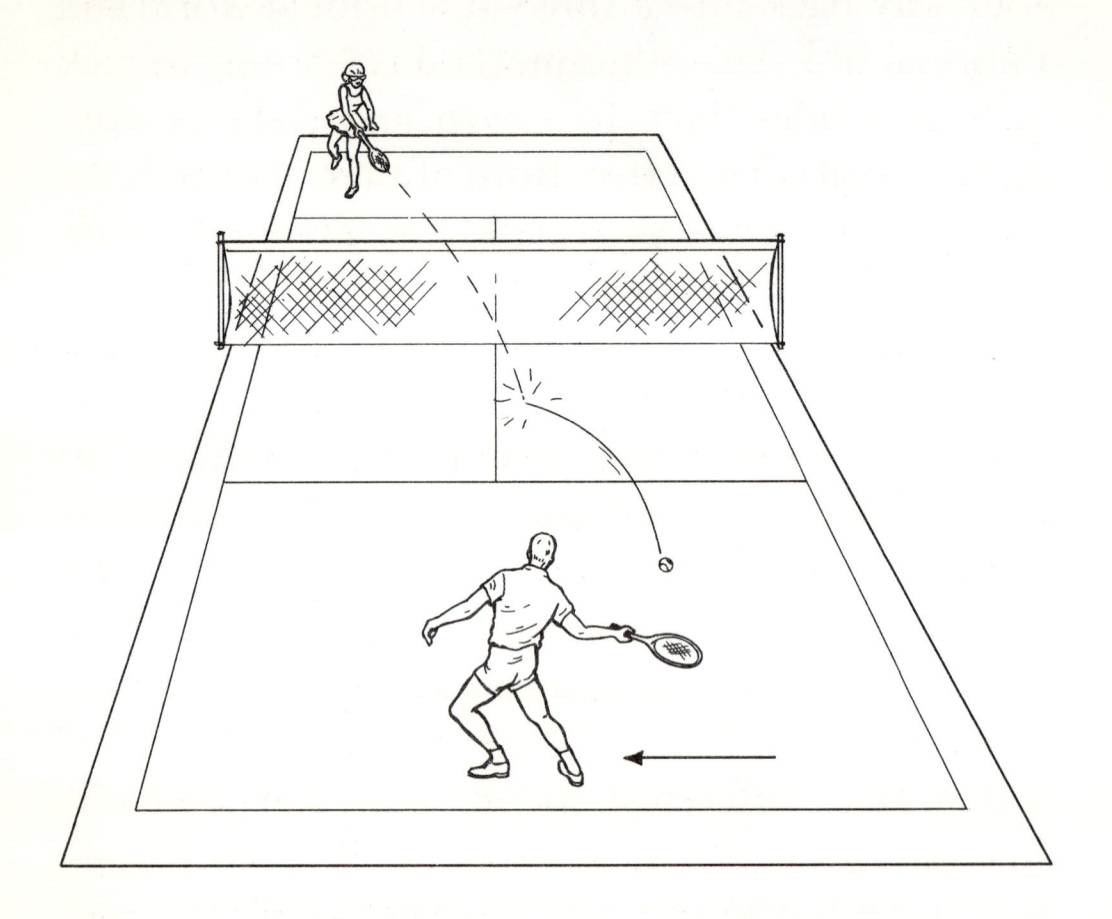

Putting the relative motion principle to work, the player above quickly shifts his position so that the ball doesn't come directly at him. The angle thus created improves his judgment.

Is there anything you can do to remedy this situation? Certainly. Shift your position. With one quick movement you can place yourself off to the side, creating the angle of approach your brain needs to compute the ball's relative motion (relative in relation to you). Your chances of whacking the ball with the center of your racket have now improved a thousandfold. You have used a technique. You have met a challenge.

In the absence of binocular vision, relative motion is going to be your prime visual tool in the highly mobile world of driving, flying, boating, skiing, skating and skin diving, and in occupations involving moving objects or vehicles. Knowledge of how to create it when it doesn't occur by itself can hasten your return to your favorite sport or the wheel of your car.

One illustration will suffice to show the extreme importance of developing this skill in driving. Every motorist is familiar with the driver who starts to pass you in the left lane, but then slows down and drives neck and neck with you for a long distance. This situation, irksome under the best conditions, is extremely irritating to the one-eyed driver. Even though both cars are traveling at highway speed, the relative motion between them is zero. This means that the one-eyed driver has very little in the way of clues to the distance between the two cars.

What's the prescription here? Change speed. Go a

little faster or a little slower than he does. The result is relative motion and a much improved ability to judge the distance between the two cars. It's often that simple to sharpen your depth perception and maneuver yourself out of danger.

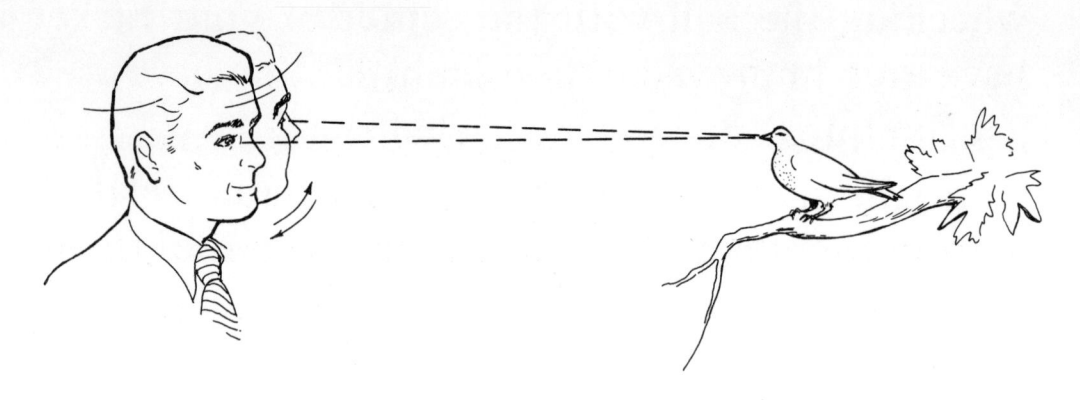

A quick side movement of your head will give two slightly different views of an object. This simulation of binocular vision creates a sense of perspective, especially at close range.

When viewing a stationary object at short range, one very effective way to produce something akin to relative motion is to move your head quickly to one side. This not only creates a slight shift of the object against its background (as did the up-and-down head movement described earlier in this chapter), it also gives you two slightly different views of the same object in such rapid sequence that the brain can interpret them much the same as it would a double image produced by two eyes.

I find this rapid head movement one of the

handiest tricks for improving distance judgment up to several feet. And while I wouldn't advise you to become a self-conscious swivelhead, I would suggest that you use your normal head movements as fully as possible to give your world a third dimension.

PERSPECTIVE

We turn to the world of art for other important methods of improving depth perception. In their endless quest for ways of depicting a three-dimensional world on a two-dimensional canvas, painters long ago came up with several techniques which can be equally useful to you in reverse—that is, in trying to convert your relatively flattened out world back into 3-D. All these techniques can be lumped under the general term "perspective."

Let's stand at a window—preferably one commanding a view—and ask the great Leonardo da Vinci to join us. Leonardo's descriptions of how he used light color and shadow to gain realism and depth in his immortal paintings have much to teach us. With the old master's help, we notice three important facts about the scene outside out window:

1. Objects in the foreground take up more of the window's space than objects of the same size in the distance. Automobiles, which are fairly standardized in size, are a good gauge of this. Leonardo

37

calls this phenomenon "diminishing perspective."

2. Colors are bolder and brighter in the foreground. In the distance they become softer and muted. By the same token, shadows of nearby objects are sharper and darker. The artist calls this "color perspective."

3. Finally, objects in the distance tend to blur, while those in the foreground are more clearly defined—the "vanishing perspective."

These observations are as precious to the one-eyed person as they are to the painter, for each of them can be translated into improved depth perception. It's a process you can hasten by consciously applying your attention to it—and as a fringe benefit you'll find the world a far more fascinating place to view.

While the rules of perspective are simple, their application to a given scene is sometimes tricky. An automobile right in front of you takes up much more of your field of vision than it does two blocks away. But since you already know its *size,* you can use its *apparent* size to estimate its distance from you.

If you know the *distance* of an object from you—for instance, if you see a round object bobbing in the water at the end of a pier whose length is familiar to you—it's not hard to estimate the round object's size. But if neither distance nor size are known to you, you'll look for other clues.

A principle used extensively in flying and boating can be extremely useful in such situations. Suppose, while you're sailing a boat on a straight course, you see another boat (of unknown size at an unknown distance) moving on a path that will eventually cross yours. Seasoned pilots warn their students to "beware of a flyspeck on the windshield that doesn't move but just grows!"

The thing to watch for is the angle of the other boat's path in relation to you. If the angle changes, and continues to change, the boat will pass clear. Beware if there's no change in angle.

This navigating technique, developed for normally sighted persons, is even more useful to the person with only one eye.

9
PITFALLS AND BOOBY-TRAPS

If your experience is anything like mine when you return to your everyday environment after the loss of an eye, you'll feel suddenly beset with pitfalls and booby traps of all descriptions and on every side. Identifying each one is half the battle; developing a technique to cope is the other half.

Nearly all the troubles you're likely to get into are traceable to two factors: loss of depth perception and reduction in field of vision caused by the existence of your nose. In the previous chapter we discussed some tricks for regaining depth perception in given situations. But the only way to cope with the cutoff on the sightless side of your nose is to develop the habit of looking around—*before* you leap. This means that you will go through life using your neck a lot more than you formerly did.

What follows is a rundown of some specific situations that can bring you bumps, jolts, embarrassments, bruises and even more serious griefs if you aren't ready for them—along with a specific antidote for each.

SHAKING HANDS

Of all my early experiences in adaptation to one-eyed vision, none caused more chagrin than reaching out to grasp a friendly hand and closing my fingers on thin air—and none is more easily avoided.

The point to remember is that you don't have to know exactly how far you are from the object you're reaching for in order to connect with it. It's not so much a question of distance judgment as it is of alignment.

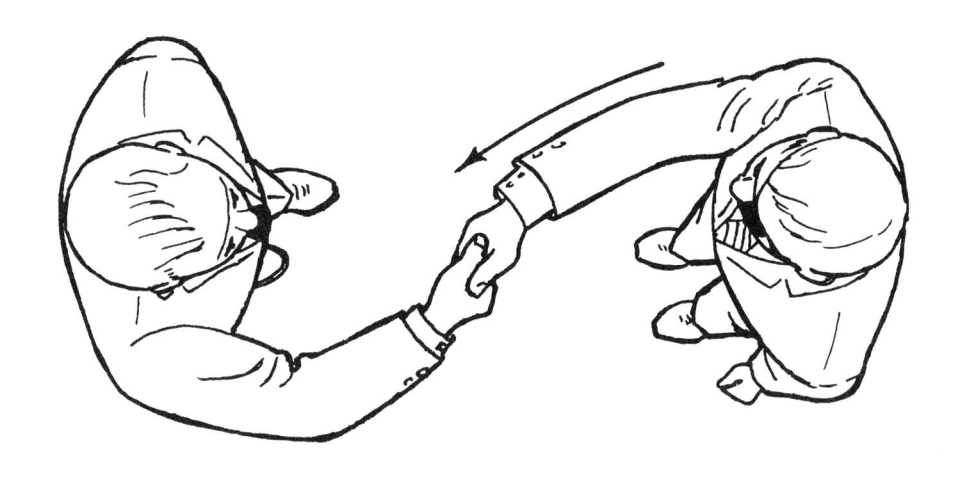

You should have little or no trouble in making contact with an object if you first remember to line up with it and then simply keep on extending your arm and hand until you touch it.

To perform this simple act with complete confidence, simply move your hand in a direct line toward the hand you wish to shake—and keep on moving until you connect. The technique, of course, is equally useful in reaching for a doorknob, a hanger in a closet, a book in a bookcase or a glass of water on a table.

POURING

The distance judgment required to pour accurately from one container (e.g., a martini pitcher) into another (e.g., a cocktail glass) comes with a

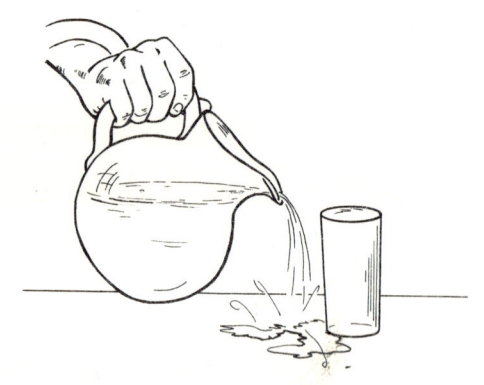

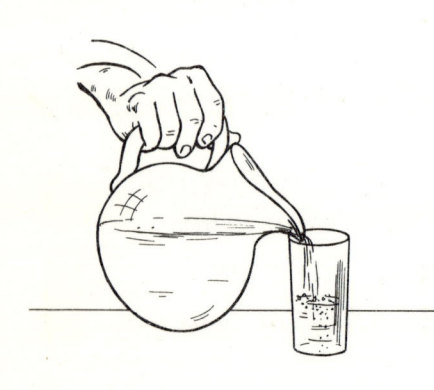

Experience will bring distance judgment necessary to pour from one container to another without missing. Until then, pour with the upper container touching the rim of the lower.

little experience. But until then it's surprisingly easy to miss your aim completely.

If you want to avoid the kind of spillage I was constantly apologizing for in my early days out of the hospital, here's a childishly simple yet sure technique: place the spout or lip of the upper container right down over the rim of the lower one so that they actually touch, then pour with abandon—you can't miss! By resting the neck of your sugar spoon on the edge of your coffee cup in the same manner, you can make sure that *all* the sugar gets into the coffee.

THE COLLISION COURSE

"I'm forever bumping into people," is one of the most common complaints of the newly one-eyed. You'll find these collisions nearly always occur when you make an abrupt turn toward the side on which your vision is partly cut off, that is, into the blind spot you checked only a moment ago and found empty.

Moral: "A moment ago" simply won't do. Check that blind spot the very instant you're ready to make your turn. That way no Sneaky Pete will take you by surprise.

The habit of checking probably won't "set" until you've had quite a few bumps. But cultivate it carefully in all situations that involve change of direction—particularly where safety is involved, as

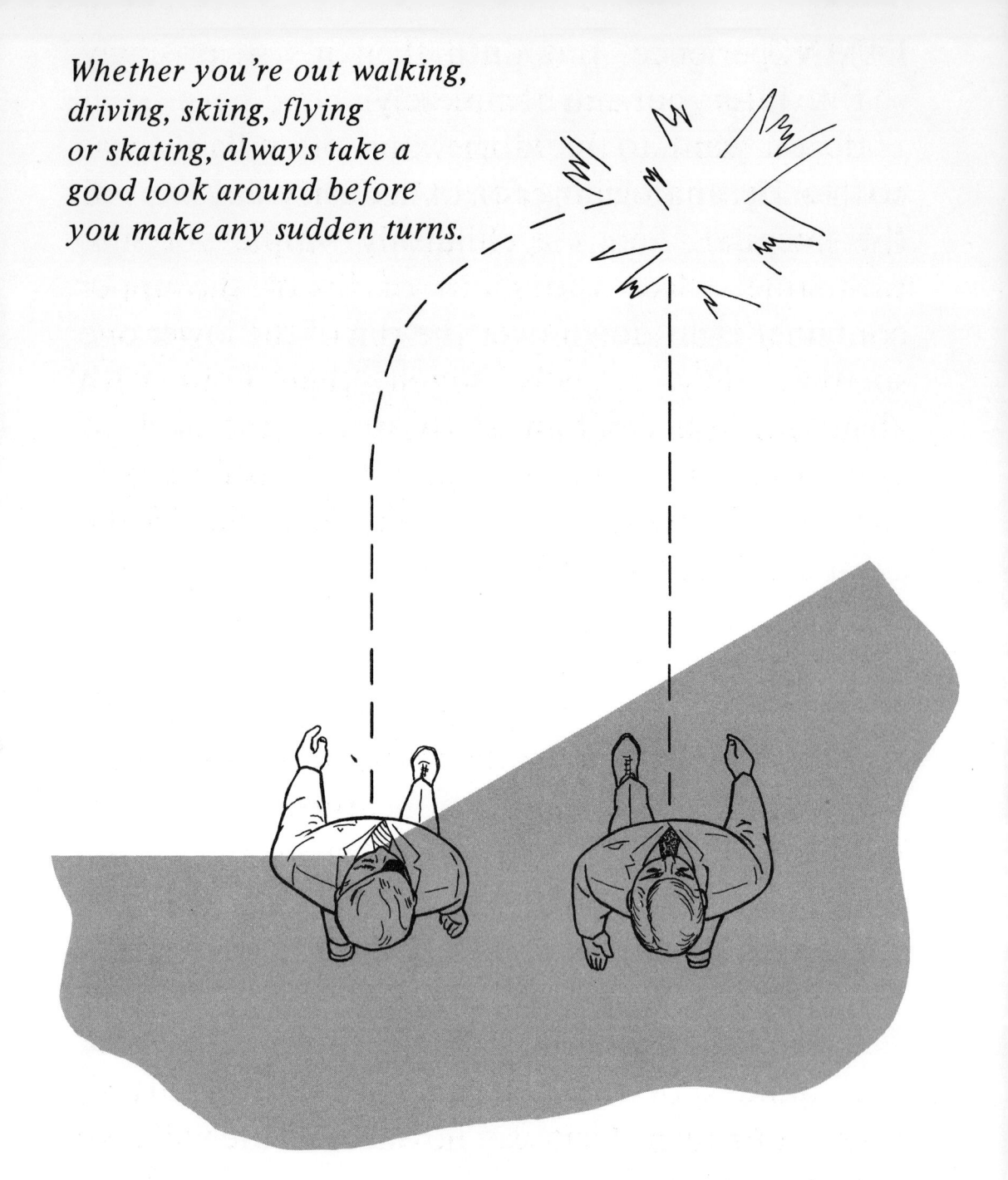

Whether you're out walking, driving, skiing, flying or skating, always take a good look around before you make any sudden turns.

in swimming, skiing, riding, skating or boating, and most especially in driving and flying. Before you change lanes on the highway, take a *very* good look around to make sure some Volkswagen hasn't crept up just outside your field of vision.

44

DINING

I've often noticed that a lefthanded person will choose a seat at the table where he won't tangle with a righthanded person when they start to eat. In the same manner—when it doesn't violate protocol or my hostess' careful seating arrange-

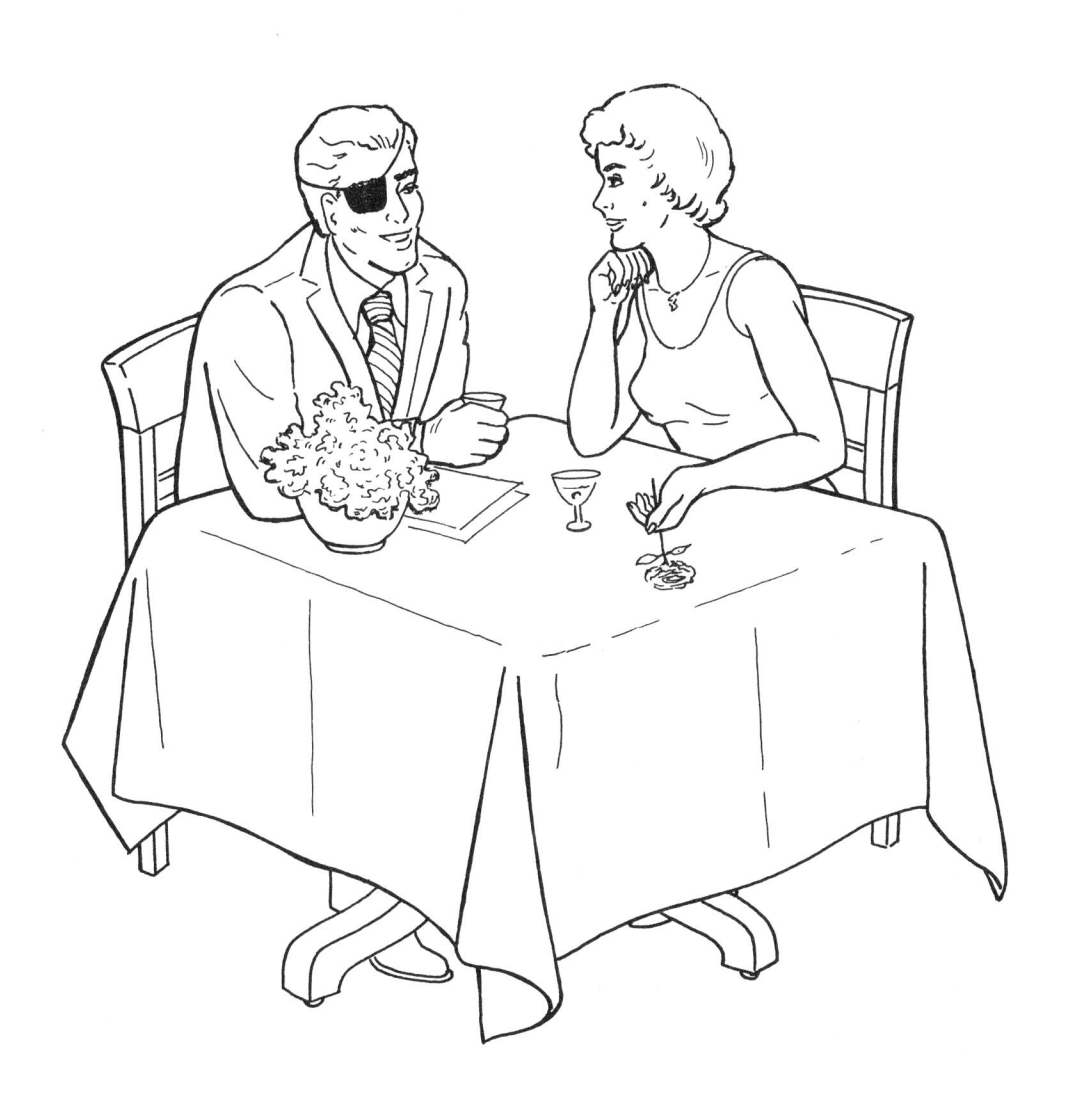

When dining, remember to choose a place at the table that favors your good eye, and watch out for waiters serving on your sightless side.

ments—I choose a seat that I hope will favor my good eye.

I find that if I'm required to keep up a conversation with a partner on my right, which happens to be the side of my visual cutoff, the excessive amount of head twisting involved can be not only tiring but annoying. A charming dinner partner may be worth the extra effort, but if you can make prior arrangements to favor your good side, everyone will be happier.

And remember that the choice of the right seat doesn't always eliminate other dining dangers. If the meal is being served by a waiter or waitress—especially a skilled, *unobtrusive* one—he may be at your sightless side the very moment you least expect him. A few bad experiences with well-trained waiters taught me to take a deliberate look to the right before making any unusual gestures in that direction.

You should be luckier, being forewarned.

STAIRWAYS

Whether you're going up or down, *watch that last step!* Viewed with one eye, it may blend right into the floor above or below it—especially if it has the same carpeting or finishing treatment. In either direction, it's all too easy to assume that you've taken the last step and start walking away, only (jolt!) to discover that there was one more.

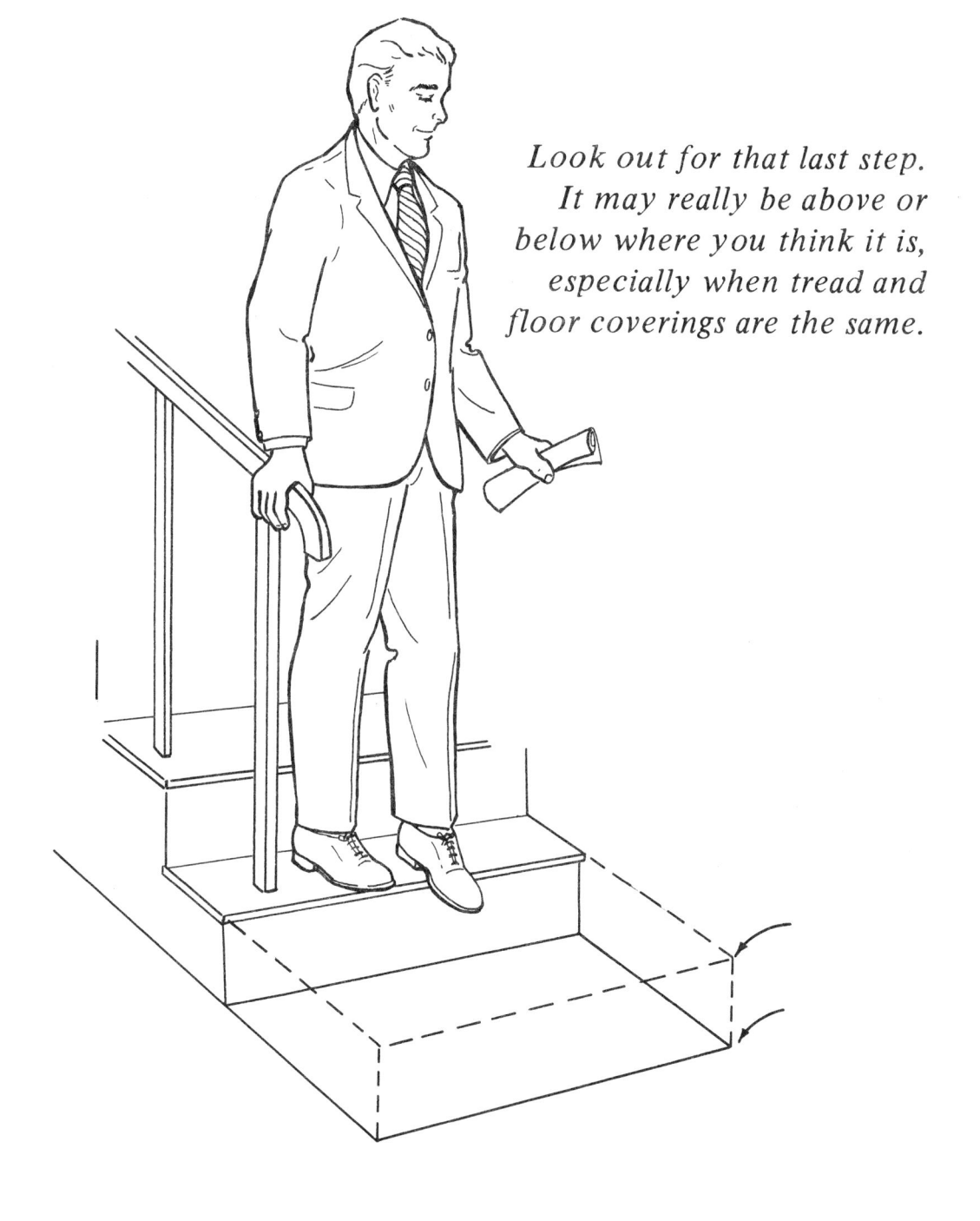

Look out for that last step. It may really be above or below where you think it is, especially when tread and floor coverings are the same.

This illusion can be particularly dangerous for the elderly. But anyone who has lost his binocular vision should take that last step gingerly—feeling ahead with his toe and keeping one hand on the handrail.

CURBS

A close relative to that last step of the stairway, the curb can be even more treacherous. As you'll quickly discover, curbs show surprisingly nasty variations in height from one street corner to the next. There are no handrails to hold onto, and a single misjudgment could easily jolt you into the middle of traffic.

After this dire warning, I'm sure you'll immediately start practicing the simple trick I've discovered for estimating the height of a curb without

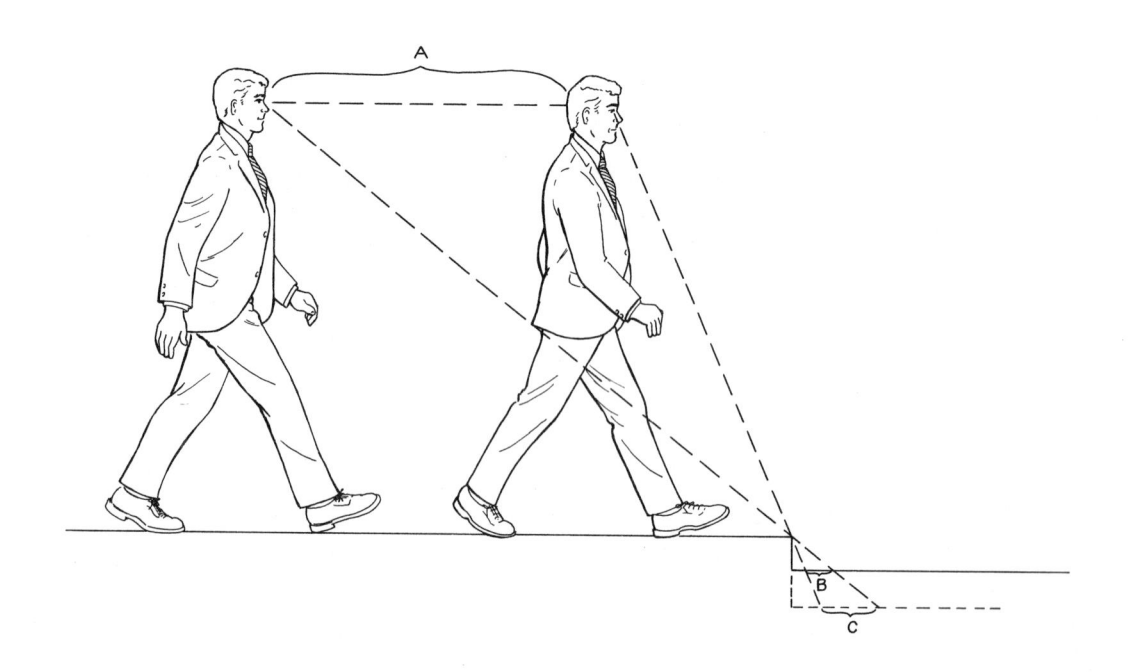

Use the curb edge as a reference point to judge curb height. For a low curb, segment B will be short compared with C for a higher curb.

benefit of binocular vision. It uses the same principle of relative motion that we've already explored.

As you approach the street, keep your eye on the edge of the curb so you can observe its relative movement against the background of the street's surface. The higher the curb, the faster will this relative motion appear and the more street paving will it bring into view. Your brain will have no trouble at all computing these factors, along with your walking speed, and will send you a message telling you just how deep a step to take when you hit the street.

With a little practice (and I suggest that you do your *initial* practicing in a safe place) the technique will become so much a part of your adaptation that you won't even have to think about it. It will serve you equally well wherever you have to judge the distance between two horizontal surfaces. Once you've learned it, you need have no qualms about accepting an invitation to go mountain climbing or go spelunking.

CROSSING STREETS

Now I've got you to the curb, I'd better alert you to the dangers out there on the street itself. You're well aware, I'm sure, of the dangers traffic poses for a pedestrian with two good eyes. But the special hazard for the one-eyed is the car that comes from an unexpected quarter on your wrong side. The only way to cope, of course, is to develop the habit of looking both ways *at the very last moment*—and particularly on the side with limited peripheral vision.

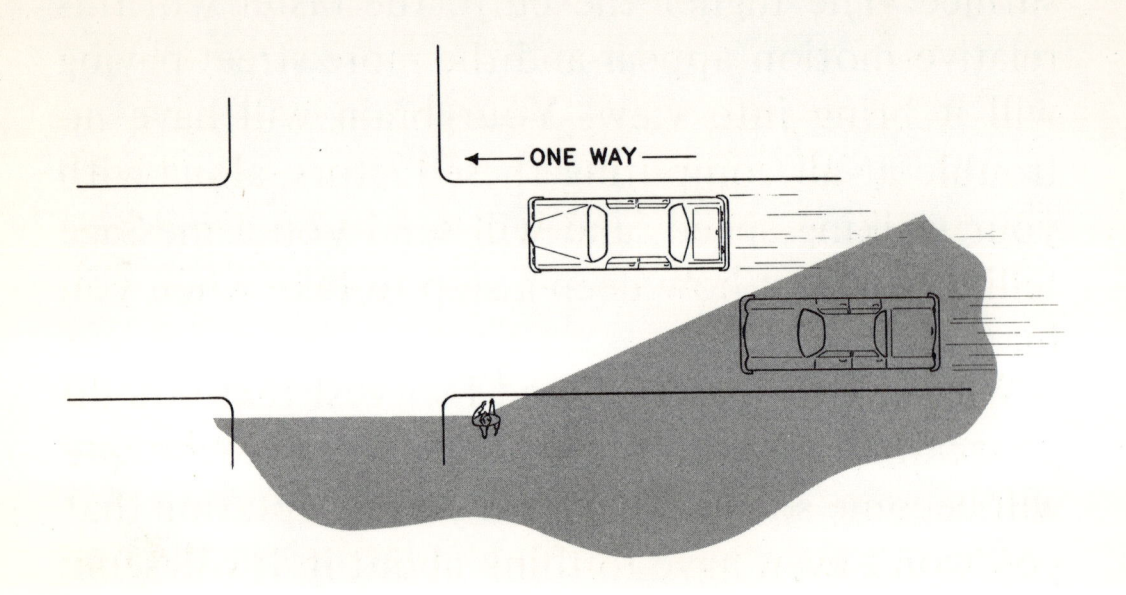

Always be sure to take a good look both ways before stepping off any curb into the street. But as illustrated above, particular care is necessary when crossing one-way streets.

Beware of intersections where cars are permitted to make right and left turns. That car that wasn't signaling when you last looked may be turning anyway. Even if you have the right of way, the driver may assume that you'll see him and step aside.

A special danger is the one-way street you haven't been alerted to—especially if you have a right-side visual cutoff and the traffic is moving from that quarter. If you assume you're crossing a normal two-way street and look first to your left, you might easily step off the curb into the path of a car bearing down on your right.

A particularly vicious form of this danger awaits the one-eyed visitor to Great Britain and other countries where motorists still drive on the left. Busy crossings in London have signs on the pavement reminding you to "Look to Right," but elsewhere in this nation it's all too easy to step into a lethal situation.

Once you've lost your binocular vision, the best advice anyone can give you for crossing streets is: *Use your head.*

THREADING A NEEDLE

This simple act, when first attempted with one eye, can seem as exasperatingly difficult as trying to pin the tail on the donkey with both eyes blindfolded. Don't rage, don't despair. Here's a technique that works:

1. Cut the thread at an angle with a very sharp pair of scissors or a razor blade. Make sure there's no fuzz on the end. The thread will

now have a definite point at the end you've cut.
2. Sharpen that point by moistening it and drawing it between your fingers.
3. Hold the needle toward the light and wipe the point of the thread back and forth across the needle, slowly withdrawing it until it just doesn't touch. The trick is to get the point as close as possible to the eye before the final step.
4. Now center the point of the thread on the eye of the needle and push it through.

However, a simple needle-threading device such as you can buy in any five-and-ten-cent store (below), will make the job considerably easier—

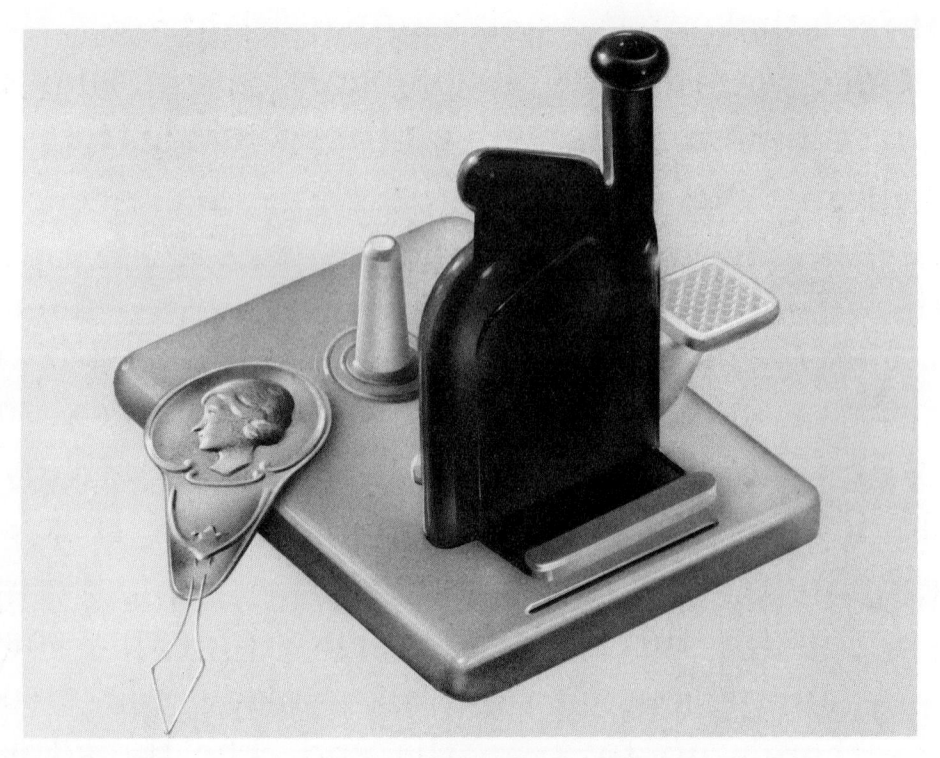

Two common needle-threading devices.

especially if you also apply the techniques listed above.

SHOOTING

Firing a rifle or shotgun is a sport that normally calls for the use of only one eye. Yet paradoxically it poses a problem for some marksmen who suddenly find themselves with only one eye.

The reason is not abstruse. It lies in the fact, already discussed, that righthanded people are right-eyed, and lefthanded people left-eyed. This creates no problem with side arms—only with guns that must be braced against the shoulder. The marksman with right-side dominance normally holds the stock against his right shoulder, places his left foot forward and sights with his right eye.

If he loses that eye, he's in for a shock the next time he tries to aim a gun. He finds that if he takes his normal stance and holds the weapon against his right shoulder, the gunstock prevents his left eye from lining up with the sights. And a person who loses a dominant left eye, of course, faces the same problem in reverse.

The most common, perhaps the best way, to cope with this problem (though I'll give you some alternatives in Chapter 12) is "switching." This means simply reversing your stance and holding the gun against the other shoulder so as to line up the sights with your good eye.

The first time you try this, everything will feel all wrong. Your scores will show a dramatic drop, particularly if you're shooting at a live or moving target. It'll never work, you'll quickly conclude. Yet many persons who'd rather switch than fight have with persistence brought their scores back up to their old levels.

One enthusiastic advocate of switching is my friend Jack Fletcher, a photographic specialist with the National Geographic Society. An avid skeet fan, Jack had been shooting for years without ever having achieved a perfect score. Then he lost his dominant right eye and had to find an instructor to teach him how to shoot off his left shoulder. The training was so successful that Jack has since shot not one but several perfect scores.

One precaution: Guns with automatic ejection devices are designed to eject the shells away from the person who is firing—and most of them are for shooting off the right shoulder. Switching could cause the shell to fly toward you and create a hazard. Be sure to keep this problem in mind when you select your firearms.

EXERCISE

Practically all the skills called for in the simple acts of everyday living with one eye can be sharpened by exercising with a ball. Simply bouncing a ball off a wall for a few minutes each day or playing catch with a friend can improve your visual skills enormously. So can any of the ball games like tennis, baseball or basketball.

All these activities demand accommodation and call for judgment of angle size, distance, relative motion and timing. And all the gains you make in these activities can be carried over into your daily routines.

10

IN THE DRIVER'S SEAT

There is no reason why, under normal circumstances, you can't learn or continue to drive with only one eye. (Chapter 15, "Driver and Pilot Licensing Standards," will give you specific information concerning licensing requirements in each of the United States.) But there are a few situations in driving that you may find a bit bothersome and which will require some special attention.

I'm sure you'll have no more trouble than I did on the open highway. Actually most of your visual problems will be on narrow, crowded streets, where you're driving slowly and trying to judge distances on either side of you.

One difficult feat, until you're accustomed to monocular vision, is threading your way through a narrow lane between parked cars without scraping any paint off them. Three ways to handle this (in increasing order of difficulty) are:

1. Follow the car ahead of you. With this "guinea pig" to tell you if it's safe to proceed, you'll have no problem (unless you're driving a

Cadillac and following a Volkswagen).
2. If there's no car ahead of you, then *press your passenger into service* to assure clearance on the right while you concentrate on the left.
3. If you have no passenger, *look ahead to make sure you have adequate clearance, and concentrate all your attention to driving close to the line of cars on your left*—with your head out the window if necessary.

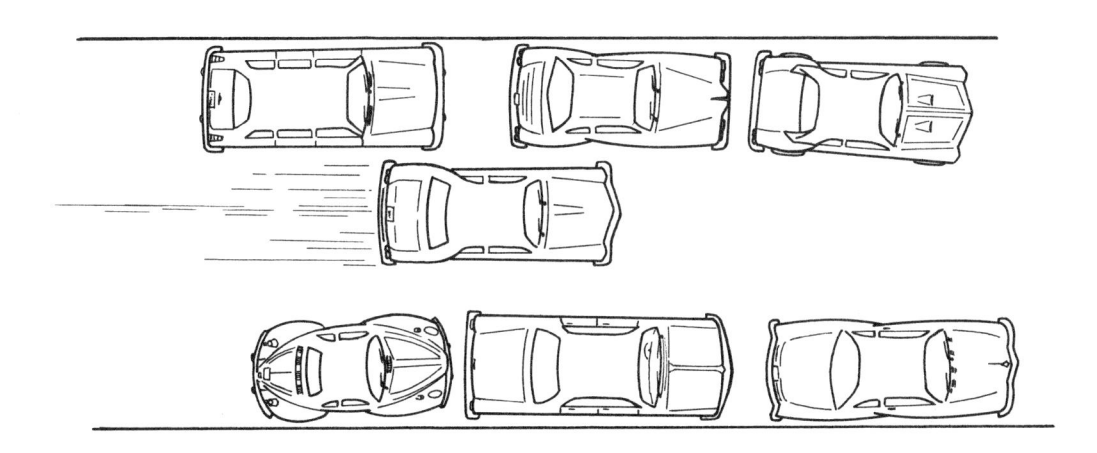

Until you get used to monocular vision you'll probably have trouble working your way between parked cars on a narrow street. Tip: Keep left!

A more nerve-twanging variant of this is the narrow two-way street where you have to make room for an oncoming car without touching the

57

cars parked to your right. Your three alternatives in this problem are:

1. Drive close to the center line so as to leave plenty of room between yourself and the parked cars without going onto his half of the street.
2. If there is no center line, *project a "mental" one onto the street* and try to use it the same way.
3. If this proves too difficult, *stop your car at the widest available space* and wait for him to pass.

Auto safety engineers could make a real contribution by requiring that corner posts on all new cars be designed to minimize visual obstruction. The wide posts so popular on some cars today can block out an astonishingly large swath of the scene to the rear, even for a driver with good binocular vision. When sight is limited to one eye, the problem is severely aggravated, and the only antidote I know is a limber neck. Frequent head movements will enable you to see around the obstruction and avert any compromise with safety.

PARKING

One of the things you sooner or later must learn is to accept your limitations. If you know what you can't do, you may save yourself a lot of pain and frustration by trying to avoid certain situations altogether.

Consider parking. Before my accident I prided myself on my deftness in parking an automobile. So it took some ulcerating experimentation to convince me that I'm just not adept anymore. I find that maneuvering my car into a tight space in a parking lot between two other cars—and knowing that the slightest bump can result in costly damage, thanks to incredibly bad auto design—is often more aggravation than it's worth.

If there's a passenger with me, I have no hesitancy about putting him to work to help me clear the other cars. When I'm alone, I sometimes get out of my car to survey the situation and plan my maneuvers with precision. But more often, if there's time, I'll try to find a wider slot or even go considerably out of my way to find a spot I can get into and out of with ease.

Maybe parking will be a snap for you. I often marvel at the aplomb of a garage attendant in my office building. While wearing a patch over one eye, this young man races the cars through underground labyrinths, jockeying this one and that one from rear to front, all with the greatest assurance and enjoyment. Whether his monocular vision has anything to do with the dents and scratches customers claim they sometimes find on their cars, I'm not in a position to say. But I wish I knew the secret of his assurance.

I *have* developed a trick or two for snuggling into

59

your own garage without hitting the rear wall. Try turning on the headlights, even in the daytime, and watching the patterns the beams make on the wall as you approach it. In no time you'll be able to come within an inch and not hit. At night you can also back in and use the backup lights in the same manner.

Another very simple and effective aid is a short strip of tape pasted vertically on the sidewall of the garage adjacent to your good eye to mark your stopping point. I find that my garage parking using this technique is much more uniform and accurate than that of other drivers in my family who rely solely on depth perception.

11

THE ACTIVE LIFE

Anyone who feels that the loss of an eye marks the end of sports for them should consider the case of Sue Moran, radio and television personality, fashion model, committeewoman and mother of six. Mrs. Moran's 10-year bout with a corneal inflammation ended, in 1965, with the loss of her right eye.

"It hasn't changed my life," she says. "I'm still doing all the things I enjoy and still coping with the endless demands of a large family and a country home."

Among the things Mrs. Moran enjoys is riding in such competitions as the International Horse Show in Washington, where she has won a reputation for her skill in the vanishing art of riding sidesaddle. She also enjoys fox hunting, beagling, swimming, skiing and bird watching—all sports that make heavy demands on visual perception and judgment.

Because the speeds involved demand lightning judgments, skiing would seem to require the ultimate in visual perception. Yet ski-jumper Jerry Martin from Minnesota has proved that top-level, competitive skiing is really possible with one eye.

Martin lost the sight in his right eye in September, 1971, when a nail he was pounding into brick bounced back and struck his cornea. Although he expects eventually to regain normal sight with a transplant and a contact lens, he has done some amazing things in the meantime. Six weeks after his injury he was jumping again. And he was doing it so well that by January, 1972, he won the tryouts for the U.S. Olympic Team with a leap of 318 feet. (He failed to win a medal at the Olympics, but he did place higher than any other American.)

Commenting on his winning tryout performance, Martin said: "My doctor told me depth perception would be the biggest problem. In ski jumping you need it for taking off and for landing, but you're only affected at a distance of about 10 feet. I've been jumping a long time and I land more by feel than by sight so I wasn't worried about that. I wanted to prove to myself that I could keep jumping with one eye. That actually gave me a little extra push."

In contrast, Sandy Duncan, brilliant TV comedy star who lost the sight in one eye, gave a Life Magazine reporter an hilarious account of her efforts to learn to ski. Time after time, while standing and talking with her instructor, she would suddenly find herself starting to slide down the slope: "Finally we figured it out. Because of this eye thing I can't determine the fall line. I would think I was exactly on the perpendicular when in fact I was headed straight down the slope." But with the same determination she's shown in coping with her handicap, Miss Duncan added, "I'll learn."

As you test yourself out in the sports that have always given you pleasure, there are a few important physical and psychological factors to keep in mind. From a purely physical standpoint, those sports in which the motion takes place in two dimensions rather than three—bowling, billiards, croquet and shuffleboard, for example—will be the easiest to remaster. Since the object of play is confined to a single plane, the simple visual judgments demanded in these sports can be handled with one eye just about as well as with two.

In three-dimensional sports, where monocular vision presents more of a challenge, your difficulties will be determined by a whole complex of factors. A basketball, for instance, will be easier to manage than a handball; you'll miss less often with a racket than with a bat; a fast game like jai alai will come a lot harder than a slower one like badminton.

But given the right psychological set, none of the sports are beyond the capabilities of the person who has lost an eye. Nor is there any reason to give up those that have always brought you enjoyment.

The main thing to remember is that some sports call for a longer period of relearning than others, and that during this period you're competing only with yourself.

This psychological stance may be a little harder to acquire in such games as tennis and baseball, where the emphasis seems to be entirely on beating an adversary. If you find any of these too frustrating, why not try making your comeback, initially, in sports that have well established handicaps, like golf? Or those that pit you against your own record, like archery or rifle practice? Or those that you can engage in purely for fun and exercise—as well as for competition, when you want it—like water sports?

Water sports, in fact, have so much to recommend them to the newly one-eyed that I would like to discuss a few of them individually.

SWIMMING

This most popular of all water sports is virtually unaffected by the limitations of monocular vision. And this is true not only of surface swimming, but of underwater swimming with snorkel or scuba equipment.

Underwater distance judgments are difficult even with normal eyesight because water bends the light differently from the way air does. Moreover, most underwater masks limit the field of vision so much that it makes no difference whether you have one eye or two.

So if this activity appeals to you, it's one of the best ways to get back in the swim.

DIVING

You'll encounter no special problems here either, unless you wear an artificial eye. The sudden pressure when you strike the water, particularly in a high dive, can dislodge the prosthesis. A pair of underwater goggles is the answer. Make sure the lenses are high-impact and shatter-resistant to safeguard your good eye.

FISHING

Although some distance judgments are involved in casting a lure, the distances are beyond the range where binocular vision is any real help. Out on the Bahama flats I've watched my one-eyed friend Clarke Daniel drop his shrimp-baited hooks time after time directly in front of bonefish with all the skill and precision of a native bonefish guide.

The chief danger is having a wild cast put a hook into an eye that wasn't meant for it. Lewis Williams Douglas lost an eye this way while serving as U.S. ambassador in Britain. With only one good eye, you simply can't afford to take that chance, so always wear protective glasses with high-impact, shatter-resistant lenses.

WATER SKIING AND SURFING

These sports, though difficult in themselves, pose absolutely no special problems for the one-eyed individual.

SAILING

Just a few points for the newly monocular to remember. The danger in jumping from dock to boat and vice versa can be lessened by following the sailor's advice of "one hand for the boat."

A useful device for all skippers, but particularly the one-eyed, is the "telltale"—bits of yarn placed on the shrouds or at the luff to indicate the relative direction of the wind and help obtain the proper trim.

A monocular for checking distant buoys and an illuminated magnifier for reading charts at night are also useful. A "monkey fist," or padded weight at the end of a small line, can improve your accuracy when you toss a line to shore or to another boat. Ingenious devices like these can more than compensate for the limitations of monocular vision. In the next chapter, we will talk about other devices you'll find helpful.

12
GIMMICKS AND GADGETS

How do you turn a handicap into an asset?

One way is by taking full advantage of all the marvelous gadgetry created to compensate—even overcompensate—for every imaginable deficiency. Many persons deprived of binocular vision have found that one eye plus a gadget plus a little practice results in a better performance than had been thought possible with two eyes unaided. So let's examine some of the aids and instruments you may find helpful.

EYEGLASSES

When you've lost one eye, it becomes imperative to protect the surviving one and to enhance its vision to the greatest practicable degree. Of course, only an eye specialist can tell you whether you need glasses and prescribe the proper corrective lens for you. But there are some special considerations you'd do well to keep in mind when you go to get his prescription filled. There've been quite a few developments in eyeglasses since Ben Franklin invented bifocals in the eighteenth century.

One of the latest and greatest improvements is the new safety standard set by the U.S. Food and Drug Administration. Under a regulation that took effect January 1, 1972, all eyeglasses, including nonprescription sunglasses, must be impact-resistant. This means that the lenses must be able to withstand the impact of a steel ball, the size of a marble, dropped from a height of 50 inches.

To meet this requirement, lenses are now made of a special plastic or of heat-hardened crown glass. Either of these materials may add to the cost of a pair of glasses, but the amount is small when compared to the added protection they give your eyes—especially if you've already used up your "spare."

Your visual field, as you know, has already been reduced, and for some activities you certainly won't want to cut it down any further. So choose eyeglass styles accordingly. Glasses with heavy frames, for instance, may be fine for reading, but they cut off so much of your field that they constitute a severe—and totally unnecessary—handicap when you're driving a car, watching a ball game or engaging in any other activity that calls for a panoramic view.

Thin-rimmed or rimless glasses cut this problem to a minimum, and a contact lens eliminates it altogether. The crescent-shaped half glasses that many people use for reading are also good in this respect, since you get an unobstructed view over the top of the lens.

There are special frames for sportsmen, featuring a headband that keeps them from being knocked off—a type appreciated by any yachtsman who has ever lost a pair of glasses overboard. (Floating frames are another solution to this problem.) Sports frames are available with cushioned nosepieces that protect both glasses and wearer from substantial shocks.

You can also choose from a wide variety of lens tints and coatings designed for special purposes. A shade of yellow, for example, is favored for shooting because it absorbs blue light, providing maximum haze penetration. Some lenses are treated so they'll darken when sunlight hits them, thus sparing the wearer the nuisance of changing glasses every time he goes out in the sun or comes back indoors.

A nonreflective coating has been developed that not only makes the wearer's eyes more visible to others, but reduces distracting reflections and ghost images for him. Because most of the light passes through the lens instead of being reflected away, the wearer gets a clearer view. Nonreflecting glasses are said to be particularly useful for driving.

The reason for mentioning these features is not to recommend that you use them, but to make you aware of them so that you can discuss your particular needs with an ophthalmologist. And remember that whatever type of glasses you're buying—whether for improved vision or protection from the sun or whatever, be sure to safeguard your single precious eye by specifying nonshatterable lenses that comply with the law.

EMERGENCY "GLASSES"

Ever get caught in front of a telephone book with no glasses to keep the print from blurring? Here's an emergency measure I picked up somewhere—and have often been thankful for ever since:

Take a small piece of cardboard or paper—a calling card is fine—and punch a tiny hole in it with a pin or a bent paper clip (the lead in an automatic lead pencil will also do nicely). Now place your eye against the hole, hold the small print about 6 inches from your eye—and read. What you've got is a lens that operates on the same principle as Grandfather's pinhole camera. You may not want to read *Gone With the Wind* this way, but it works in an emergency.

MAGNIFIERS

The loss of an eye can become much more of a problem if vision deteriorates in the surviving eye. One kind of deterioration affecting many adults is a decreasing ability to focus on near objects. In the one-eyed this can easily reach a point where even corrective glasses are inadequate for reading small print or doing close work.

A magnifying glass can often solve the problem, and there's a wide selection available, ranging from small pocket versions to large desk units. Some industrial models are mounted on stands so both hands are free to work beneath the glass.

Many units combine a magnifier and a light source, such as a flashlight behind the lens or a fluorescent tube encircling it. There are models for yachtsmen, jewelers, artists, photographers, stamp collectors and just ordinary people who want to be able to read a number in the telephone book.

RANGEFINDERS

If your camera is the kind that requires you to estimate the distance in order to focus it, by all means trade it in for one equipped with a rangefinder or a focusing viewfinder.

At critical short distances—the same that are likely to give you trouble when you've lost binocular vision—your camera requires more exact focus; and a rangefinder or a focusing viewfinder will give you far better results than you ever got by estimating, even when you had two good eyes.

Several rangefinders have recently appeared on the market that should prove useful to hunters, fishermen, yachtsmen, golfers, land estimators and others who have a need for reasonably accurate

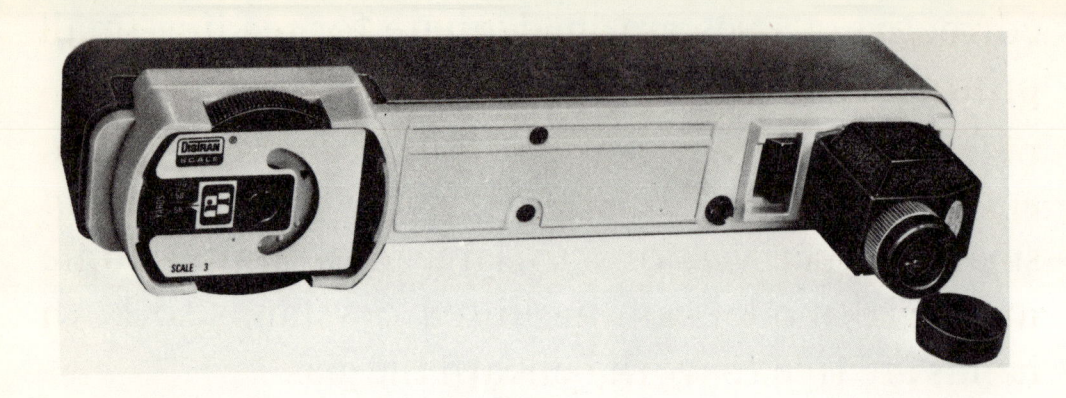

Rangefinders are invaluable aids in determining distances. The model shown here works on the stereopsis (coincidence of images) principle.

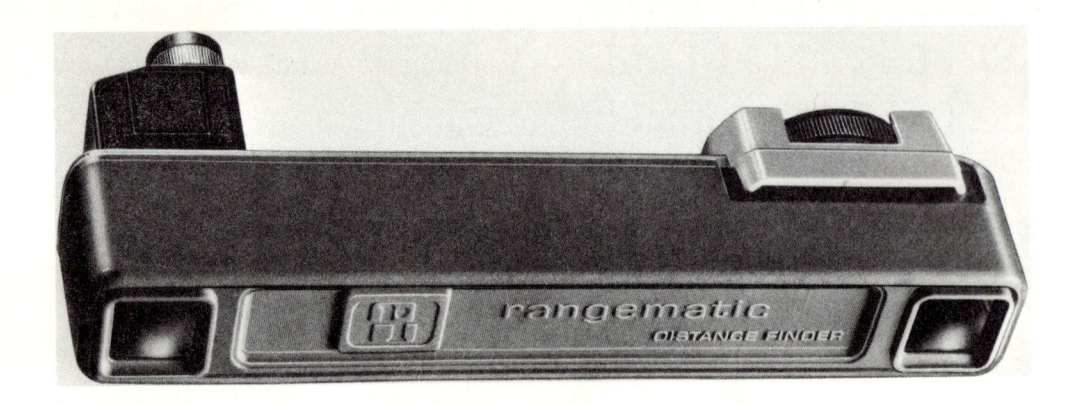

distance measurements. One of these, called the Rangematic, works on the same stereopsis principle as the camera rangefinder but has much greater spacing between the viewing lenses and hence can be used over greater distances than the camera rangefinders. If our eyes were separated by 10 inches, we would also be able to judge the distance of far objects more accurately.

The manufacturer of the Rangematic unit claims an accuracy of 95 per cent up to 500 yards and a 99 per cent accuracy at 100 yards.

Another unit, the Davis-Ordco Ranger, works on a different principle. You need only to select an object of known height or length, set two dials and read the distance from a scale. For example, knowing the height of the pin on a golf green, a player would set the dials, read off the distance and select the right club for a shot.

In golf as well as other activities requiring distance judgments, the one-eyed player is at a disadvantage only when concerned with short distances. The rangefinders described above might be highly useful to persons with normal vision.

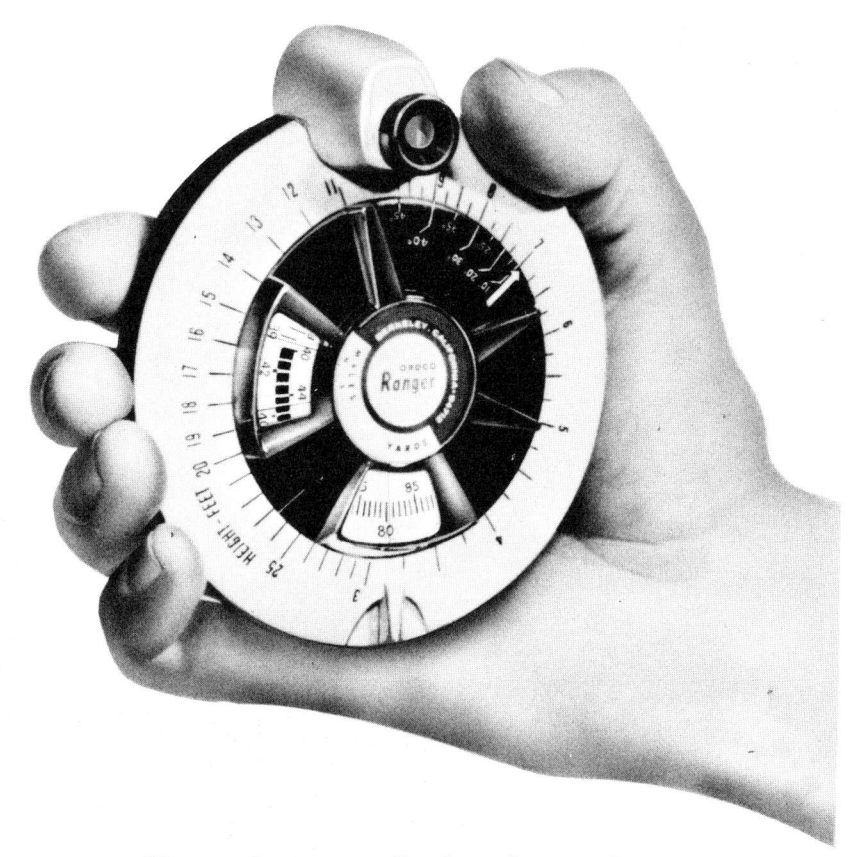

This compact, stadimetric rangefinder depends on knowing the length or height of an object.

OTHER OPTICAL AIDS

Many gadgets are available for raising your eyepower. If you shop the optical goods market, you'll find a wide variety of instruments actually designed to be used with one eye—telescopes, microscopes, loupes and monoculars, to name a few.

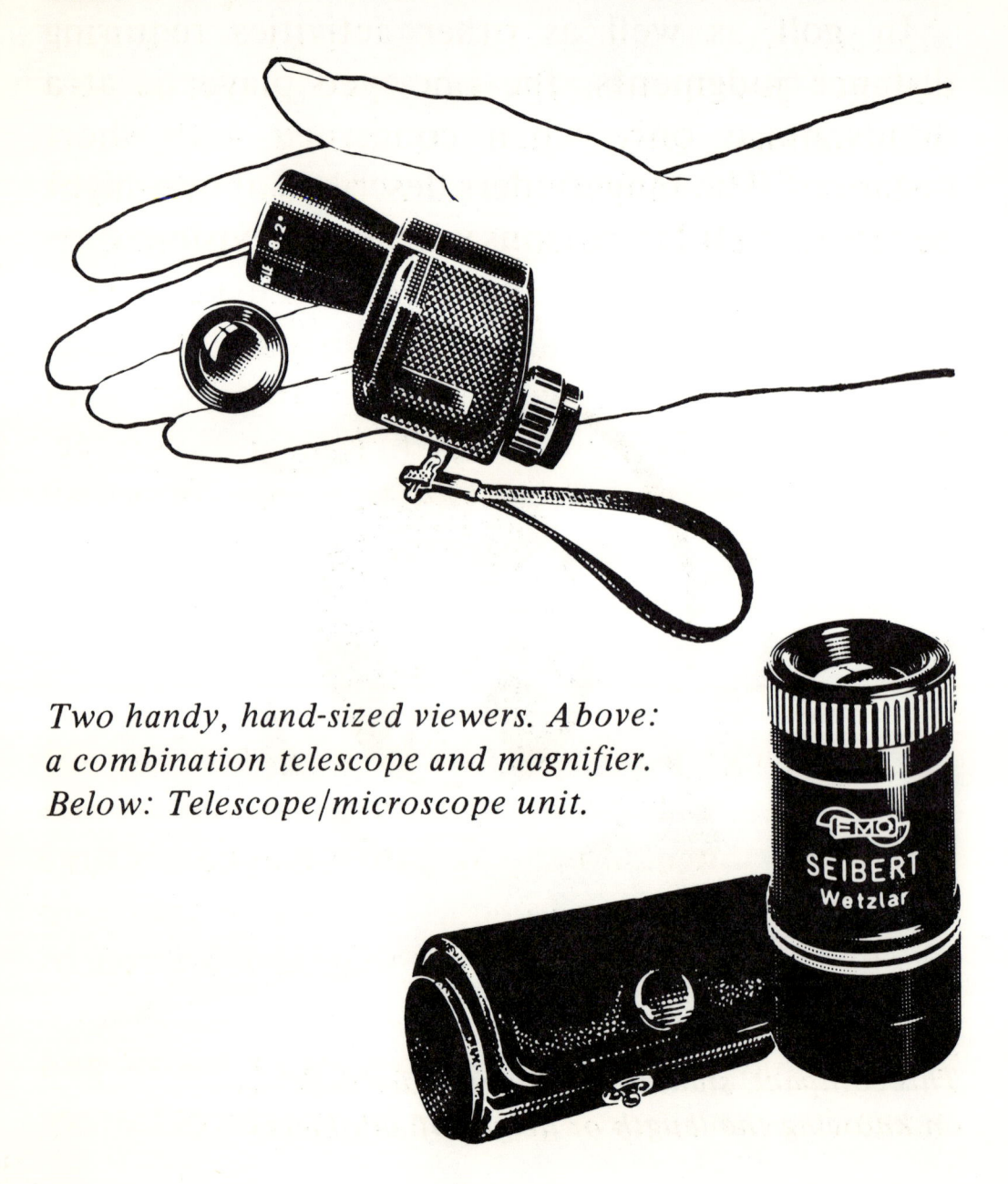

Two handy, hand-sized viewers. Above: a combination telescope and magnifier. Below: Telescope/microscope unit.

Persons with normal binocular vision sometimes have difficulty learning to use these instruments, because there's always the problem of "What'll I do with the other eye?" Students who must use single lens microscopes for long periods are taught to keep both eyes open—and it usually takes them quite a while to avoid being distracted by what the unused eye is seeing. Closing that eye for long periods, on the other hand, can become increasingly uncomfortable.

For the one-eyed there is happily no such problem. You'll find any one of these instruments easy to use at first try and, if it's well made, highly effective. Moreover, if you like this sort of thing, you can buy them in combinations to delight your gadgeteering heart—a telescope-magnifier-loupe, for instance, or a microscope-telescope-loupe—all designed to fit your already bulging pocket (if not your pocketbook).

LARGE PRINT

If you get a lot of your kicks out of reading, but find that type seems to shrink year by year so that glasses no longer do the job, then maybe it's time you tried a new approach. Here's one that you might call the mountain-to-Mohammed approach: bigger type.

A whole new world of large-print books and magazines awaits you, ranging from ancient history to modern cookbooks, from Homer to Hemingway. Children's books, maps, song sheets and crossword puzzles are now available, and new material is being added to the list all the time. Many public libraries stock a selection of large-print books. And The New York Times now publishes a weekly summary newspaper in large type. For further information about books write:

Large Print, Ltd.
505 Pearl Street
Buffalo, N.Y.
14204

For information concerning the newspaper write:

The New York Times
Large Type Weekly
Dept. 0229
220 West 43rd St.
New York, N.Y.
10036

MEASURING TOOLS

It's the little distances that get you down, remember? The inches, feet and yards. So keep an extra-generous supply of ordinary measuring tools near at hand—tape measures, yardsticks, rulers and carpenter's rules. Being forced to make exact measurements instead of guessing will bring the blessings of precision into many jobs you perhaps once didn't do nearly so neatly and nicely.

LIGHTING

I strongly believe that special kinds of lighting can do much to compensate for impairments in vision, but other than my own experience I have little evidence to back me up. Much work has been done in studying special lighting requirements of the aged, but I have found nothing directed toward the special problems of monocular vision.

Lighting for *normal* vision, by contrast, has been the subject of a great many studies. As a result of this research, illuminating engineers always strive for uniform, shadowless light wherever work is done that demands close, critical inspection.

I do a lot of close work myself, and I've found, since losing an eye, that this kind of shadowless light, such as you get from rows and rows of fluorescent tubes, is far from satisfactory for really critical tasks. I much prefer a strong, localized light source such as a small, high-intensity lamp, supplemented by a lower level of general illumination. The sharp, definite shadows produced by a high-intensity lamp can be put to excellent use in gauging depth and distance.

Let me give you an example. A small light source mounted close to the work table of a drillpress can be adjusted to cast a sharp shadow of the drill onto the work. As the drill is lowered, the shadow indicates just where the point will touch, and the work can be moved so that the point of the drill will meet its mark precisely. And this same principle can be used in the kitchen, the office, the hobby den—wherever exactness counts.

In the absence of any more scientific evidence than my own say-so, I would suggest that you experiment with various combinations of lights, adjusting the angles and distances until you find the arrangement that seems best for the task at hand.

DRIVING AIDS

Two common, inexpensive car accessories I've found very useful are a set of curb feelers and an extra side mirror. The four wire feelers attached to the sides of the car to tell you when you're within inches of the curb can take a lot of the nerve-racking guesswork out of parking and may save the one-eyed from inflicting costly scratches and dents on their cars.

A second external mirror mounted on the right side of the car can be a big help in checking your clearance on that side, particularly at slow speeds, as when you're pulling into your garage or snaking between parked cars.

A new development of special interest to the one-eyed driver has been developed by Sylvania Electric Products, Inc., but is not yet on the market. This ultrasonic device flashes a warning light on your instrument panel whenever a car tails up from behind into your right or left cutoff area. The device, which can be installed in a side mirror or in the rear light assembly, will pick up any vehicle traveling 35 miles an hour or more when it gets within 25 feet of you. It responds to the noise generated by the engines and tires of approaching cars, and can discriminate between moving vehicles and stationary objects like trees, poles and guardrails.

Sylvania hopes to make the system available as both a factory-installed item on new cars and a self-contained unit that can be installed on older ones.

GUN GADGETRY

For the serious marksman who's lost his dominant eye, the best way of regaining his skill is switching—reversing his stance and shooting from the other shoulder. But the training required for this demands considerable time and effort—more than you may wish to give it if you're just a casual, now-and-then sort of hunter or marksman like me.

An alternative way of accomplishing the same result is to use a gun with an offset stock. I experimented with one such weapon during a visit to London—a shotgun designed to be fired off the right shoulder, but with a stock that allowed enough head movement to align the left eye with the sights.

In spite of its odd appearance, I found this gun handled very naturally. I was able to shoulder, aim and fire it quite comfortably—and with no perceptible loss of skill—the very first time I tried it. In fact it seemed to be a very good solution to the problem. Such guns are made to order by Cogswell and Harrison, Ltd.

I have heard that there are also guns with offset sights designed to accomplish the same purpose as offset stocks, but my inquiries to manufacturers have failed to locate one.

In any case, it's evident that with the options available, no hunter or marksman need be afraid that the loss of an eye—even the dominant eye—will interfere with his shooting. Of course if the dominant eye is the surviving one, there's no problem whatever.

KEEPING THE GOOD EYE GOOD

13

The care and safeguarding of eyesight is of natural concern to everyone. But for the person who has lost one of his eyes, there are two special considerations. One is the question of what to do about the nonseeing eye or—if that's been removed—the empty socket. The other is the overriding importance of protecting whatever eyesight remains in the surviving eye.

To get the best advice on eye care for the one-eyed, I consulted Dr. John W. McTigue, chief of the department of ophthalmology at the Washington Medical Center and a distinguished researcher in this field. In the course of our interviews, Dr. McTigue became so enthusiastic about my project that he agreed to grace it with a foreword. The fruits of those interviews are contained in this chapter, on which Dr. McTigue has so generously collaborated.

1. THE EYE THAT WAS

If your damaged eye has been removed by surgery (enucleated), care of the remaining socket is usually very simple. Should you decide on a "glass eye" for cosmetic reasons, make sure it's well fitted by an expert; a poorly fitted shell can irritate the conjunctiva, the mucous membrane that lines the eyelid. This or any other irritation of the socket—from infections, foreign bodies, etc.—is usually not serious, provided you have it treated promptly by an ophthalmologist.

The socket may surprise you by continuing to perform many of the functions of a normal eye socket such as blinking, winking and even the shedding of tears, since the lids and tear glands are still in working order.

If you still have your nonseeing eye, the amount of follow-up medical care it needs may vary from very frequent visits to practically none, depending on what caused the loss of vision. So make certain you understand your doctor's wishes in this respect. Routine follow-up care is usual in such cases.

Be sure to report to your doctor at once any new symptoms such as pain or redness—don't wait to see what develops!

2. THE SURVIVING EYE

Don't worry about using up your "good" eye—no matter what the old wives, male and female, may tell you. Your surviving eye is quite capable of taking on by itself all the visual tasks, no matter how demanding, that were once performed by both eyes together.

If that remaining eye is normal, it probably will require only routine preventive care—an ophthalmological check-up every two years may suffice. Again, be sure to consult your own doctor about this. Moreover, you should report to him at once if you experience any new symptoms, such as redness, blurred vision, pain in the eye or headaches.

For the one-eyed person there are just a few special questions that relate to glasses, contact lenses and injuries or diseases of the eye.

GLASSES

Even small, subtle changes in vision can become important when you've lost an eye, and you'll probably be much quicker to notice them than you used to be. It may be necessary to test your eyesight for glasses more often now; some one-eyed patients need a refraction, as this test is called, as frequently as every four months.

Any blurring in vision may be a sign that you need new glasses. The conditions that cause this blurring—myopia (nearsightedness), hyperopia (farsightedness), astigmatism (distorted vision)—can generally be corrected by a compensating lens. And so can the loss of focusing power that comes with age (presbyopia). As the surviving eye loses its elasticity, a bifocal, or even a trifocal lens may become necessary to permit quick and easy shifts in focus.

One blessing of advancing years: the eye generally stabilizes at the age of 60 or 65. After that you may be relatively free of problems caused by vision changes.

Once again, please do be sure to use safety lenses in your glasses and, if you drive, to avoid heavy frames.

CONTACT LENSES

For the one-eyed person who needs a corrective lens, the contact can be an inestimable boon—provided that the fit is accurate, that medical supervision is regular and that the patient exercises good sense about wearing it.

The great advantage of the contact lens is that it provides the clearest and widest visual field possible—which, of course, is of major importance to the person whose field is already reduced by the loss of one eye.

Sometimes, as in extreme cases of myopia or hyperopia, a contact lens is the only way to compensate for the loss of side vision. This is particularly true after the removal of cataracts, when ordinary glasses provide only "tunnel vision," a condition in which side vision is very blurry or altogether absent.

INJURIES AND DISEASES

The person who has lost one eye must exercise special vigilance to prevent the development of any condition that might affect the sight of the other. Here are a few of the more common conditions to watch out for.

Injuries. No matter how trivial an injury to your remaining eye may seem to you, have your doctor examine it without delay. Only he can decide whether treatment is needed to ensure the safety of that eye.

Should you ever be so unfortunate as to suffer a major injury to your surviving eye, don't hesitate in authorizing immediate corrective treatment, no matter how hopeless you think your case may be. Saving any vestige of your vision may make the difference in the way you get around for the rest of your life.

Infections. Any redness of the eye is a signal of *some* trouble. Usually it's nothing more serious than conjunctivitis, the inflammation of the conjunctiva known as "pink eye." But don't guess at it. Get prompt diagnosis and treatment.

Glaucoma. Your doctor can detect this insidious eye disease long before it does any noticeable damage to your vision—which is one good reason why you should never neglect your regular eye examination. If it's detected early, glaucoma is no cause for the one-eyed patient to despair. Prompt treatment to arrest it, usually by regular use of eyedrops, can prevent it from making any further inroads on your vision for the rest of your life.

Cataract. This clouding of the lens occurs commonly among older people. When it reaches a point where it interferes significantly with normal visual activity, it can be removed by surgery. This is an operation you can approach with every confidence that your normal vision will be restored with glasses or a contact lens.

Detached retina. When the retina falls away from its normal position in the eye, it's as if the film were taken out of the camera; vision is lost. But with new techniques using laser beams and freezing instruments, prompt surgery is now remarkably successful in an overwhelming percentage of cases. Normal reading vision and nearly normal side vision can usually be restored.

Other, rarer, eye diseases are equally amenable to treatment or surgery. For all its apparent delicacy, the human eye really is a tough, resilient organ. It heals promptly and completely in most cases. It will work hard for you all through your life, and will probably outlast your heart, lungs and brain. If you give your remaining eye reasonable care, you should have no anxiety about its future.

It hardly seems necessary to caution anyone who has already lost an eye about guarding against accidents to the remaining eye. After all, the National Society for the Prevention of Blindness has worked for years to alert the public about eye hazards, and their advice is of special interest to the one-eyed.

The Society's recommendations are primarily concerned with wearing safety glasses, observing industrial safety regulations, and obeying safety rules pertaining to school shops and laboratories, careful attention to directions for using household cleaning products, aerosol products, insecticides, and herbicides. They particularly caution against small objects thrown up by lawn mowers.

The Society has made strenuous efforts to assure that children's playthings are safe and to urge strict adult supervision of such activities as playing dart games, BB guns, archery and chemistry sets, and missile-type toys. Fireworks, they point out, are responsible for eye injuries to many children each year.

Use of common sense and alertness to potentially hazardous situations will do much to reduce exposure to accidents. It's pleasant to believe that lightning will not strike the same object twice, but while I was still under medical care as a result of my accident, another bird—thankfully, a much smaller one—smashed against the windshield of a small aircraft in which I was again riding co-pilot.

The bird struck directly in front of my face but because of lower speeds, its lighter weight, and the grace of God, its body did not penetrate the windshield.

14

SEEING TO YOUR LOOKS

In some cases the loss of vision on one side will have no effect whatever on the appearance and it will be practically impossible for any other person to tell which is the "working eye." If you have suffered physical damage, however, or if one eye has been enucleated, or if the area around the eye has been injured in an accident, you may have some temporary problems in the way you look.

Modern eye surgery and precision fitting of a prosthesis can virtually eliminate any appearance of imbalance between the two eyes, and plastic surgery can usually repair any damages around the eye socket. So you can nearly always count on regaining a normal appearance in good time.

If the damaged eye remains, there may be some change in appearance caused by the two pupils not tracking precisely in unison. The eyes may seem perfectly aligned when looking straight ahead, but diverge a bit when the good eye glances to one side.

The effect is usually not at all displeasing. In fact, most of us are intrigued by a slight cast in a pleasant face—it seems to add a certain piquancy or individuality. Indeed, Patrick Trevor-Roper, in his book *The World Through Blunted Sight,* notes that earlier societies considered a squint a sign of godliness and beauty. He reminds us that many great artists have gone so far as to portray their subjects with a decided squint that they did not possess in real life.

What makes these observations so important is that the way you look may not be nearly as much of a handicap as the way you *think* you look to others. We all know people who become so uncomfortable under the direct gaze of another person that they'll immediately look away. This natural shyness can be terribly exaggerated for anybody who is unsure of the appearance of his eyes. A determined effort to look people straight in the eye is perhaps the best mental discipline for overcoming this self-consciousness.

"Most important," says Sue Moran, the television personality mentioned in the chapter on water sports, "is to look at things and people straight on, turning or raising the whole head and not just the eyes." That's especially important when looking up at someone from, say, a seated position.

Mrs. Moran also has a word of advice to women who may be concerned about the bright look of an artificial eye. "If you're willing to take the time," she says, "you can do a lot with makeup—especially with eye shadow—to make your two eyes look alike. False lashes have also been very useful to me in television and fashion shows—they add shadows and help soften that starry look you sometimes get from a prosthesis."

Sandy Duncan, the TV actress, also makes effective use of false eyelashes. And in an interview with Life Magazine she describes with an inimitable sense of humor the difficulty of affixing a strip of eyelashes to the lid of her functioning eye—which must be kept closed during the process.

Television viewers may recall that when she presented "Oscars" at an Academy Awards ceremony, she wore oversized, tinted glasses. Such glasses currently are highly fashionable. But for Miss Duncan they also served to soften the glare of the stage lights and to conceal the slight disparity in movement between her damaged eye and the sound one.

Some persons, including the Nobel Prize winner, Dr. Julius Axelrod, wear glasses with only one lens slightly frosted to conceal changes in appearance or movement of a damaged eye. Such a lens is particularly useful if the sightless eye remains sensitive to light.

In our times the eyepatch seems to be a symbol, not of loss, but of achievement. It endows movie stars and even comic strip characters with an indefinable charisma and is the trademark of famous persons who wear it—Moshe Dayan, for example.

For more than 20 years a succession of male models have appeared in innumerable ads wearing a patch over the right eye and looking very distinguished in their sponsor's product, a handsome shirt. The campaign has escalated an obscure Maine shirtmaking company into one of the largest organizations in the business. And one has only to wear an eyepatch himself—and to hear the murmurs of "Ah, the Hathaway Man"—to realize the strength of the identity between symbol and product.

With that campaign, many of the one-eyed suddenly found they possessed a special mystique.

Except in fairly unusual situations, anyone whose eye has been removed can expect to wear an artificial eye. Your ophthalmologist normally will recommend that an ocularist do the actual fitting. The prescription, selection, and fitting is a matter between these two specialists and they will advise you about specific care of the artificial eye and socket. But some background information may be useful.

Surprisingly, the artificial eye is a development of great antiquity, dating back at least to the fifth century B.C. Many materials, including gold, ivory, and porcelain have been used over the centuries, but a type of modern plastic is now considered most satisfactory. Plastic has a great advantage over glass in being unbreakable; furthermore, artificial eyes made of plastic can be molded to fit damaged eye sockets better than those made of glass.

Medical science eventually developed techniques for implanting artificial pupils among the muscles so that normal eye movement was restored. These techniques, however, proved also to cause new problems, particularly in maintaining proper hygiene. So the design of conventional artificial eyes has been improved to provide a satisfactory degree of eye movement. As pointed out earlier in this chapter, such movement can be greatly aided by turning or raising the head toward the subject being viewed rather than turning just the eyes.

In selecting a matching eye, it's important to rely on the advice of your ocularist rather than on your own judgment. If he recommends an eye with a pupil slightly smaller than your natural eye, it's because experience has taught him that it will reduce the tendency toward an appearance of a "stare" and so attract less attention. He may be looking for a pleasing effect rather than an exact match. So trust his skill and judgment and it will pay dividends in improved appearance.

Most artificial eyes are worn continuously, day and night, and are removed only for cleaning. Your ophthalmologist will advise you on your specific case.

When wiping your artificial eye, remember to always wipe *towards* the nose. Otherwise you may dislodge it and cause it to rotate to an incorrect position with rather bizarre results.

15
DRIVER AND PILOT LICENSING STANDARDS

"Will I still be able to drive?"

That's one of the first questions likely to be asked by the person who has lost the use of one eye. And there's no blanket answer to it, because driving regulations vary from state to state.

However, much has been done in recent years to bring state regulations into line with nationally recommended vision standards for drivers, and today all 50 states as well as the District of Columbia will license one-eyed drivers who pass their visual tests.

The accompanying table, drawn from material compiled by American Optical Corporation, shows the visual acuity standards for each state and indicates whether depth perception and visual field tests are required. These standards are for operation of private passenger cars only. The department of motor vehicles in your state can supply information for chauffeurs and bus and truck drivers.

A quick glance at the table will make plain how much licensing requirements for one-eyed drivers vary from state to state. But the standards set forth

STATE REQUIREMENTS FOR MOTOR VEHICLE OPERATORS

(As related to persons with monocular vision)
Operators of private cars—not chauffeurs

NOTE: Minimal visual acuity standards are included for persons with vision in both eyes for comparison purposes.

State	Minimum Visual Acuity Without Glasses		Minimum Visual Acuity With Glasses		Depth Perception	Visual Field
	2 Eyes	1 Eye	2 Eyes	1 Eye	Standard Test for All Licensees?	Standards Where Test Required
Alabama	20/40	20/30	20/70	20/60	Yes	—
Alaska	20/40	20/40	20/40	20/40	Yes	—
Arizona	20/40	20/40	20/40	20/40	Yes	—
Arkansas	20/40	20/30	20/50	20/40	No	110°
California	20/40	20/40	20/40	20/40	No	—
Colorado	20/40	20/40	20/40	20/40	Yes	—

State						
Connecticut	20/40	20/30	20/40	20/30	Yes	120°
Delaware	20/40	20/40	20/40	20/40	Yes	—
District of Columbia	20/40	20/40	20/40	20/40	Special cases	130°
Florida	20/40	20/40	20/40	20/40	No	—
Georgia	20/40	20/40	20/40	20/40	Yes	—
Hawaii	20/40	20/40	20/40	20/40	Yes	140°
Idaho	20/40	20/40	20/40	20/40	Yes	Standard practice
Illinois	20/40	20/40	20/40	20/40	No	—
Indiana	20/40	20/30	20/50	20/40	Yes	—
Iowa	20/40	20/40	20/40	20/40	Yes	—
Kansas	20/40	20/30	20/70	20/30	No	Standard practice
Kentucky	20/45	20/33	20/60	20/45	No	—
Louisiana	20/40	20/40	20/40	20/40	Yes	—
Maine	20/40	20/40	20/40	20/40	Yes	Standard practice
Maryland	20/40	20/40	20/40	20/40	Yes	140°
Massachusetts	20/40	20/40	20/40	20/40	No	120°
Michigan	20/40	20/40	20/40	20/40	No	140°

State	Minimum Visual Acuity Without Glasses - 2 Eyes	Minimum Visual Acuity Without Glasses - 1 Eye	Minimum Visual Acuity With Glasses - 2 Eyes	Minimum Visual Acuity With Glasses - 1 Eye	Depth Perception - Standard Test for All Licensees?	Visual Field - Standards Where Test Required
Minnesota	20/40	20/30	20/40	20/30	Yes	Standard practice
Mississippi	20/40	20/30	20/30	20/30	Yes	120°
Missouri	20/40	20/40	20/70	20/70	Yes	140°
Montana	20/40	20/40	20/40	20/40	Yes	–
Nebraska	20/40	20/30	20/40	20/30	Yes	100°
Nevada	20/40	20/30	20/60	20/50	Yes	–
New Hampshire	20/40	20/30	20/40	20/30	Yes	120°
New Jersey	20/50	20/50	20/50	20/50	No	–
New Mexico	20/40	20/40	20/40	20/40	No	–
New York	20/40	20/40	20/40	20/40	No	–
North Carolina	20/40	20/29	20/50	20/40	Optional with examiner	–
North Dakota	20/40	20/30	20/40	20/30	No	Optional with examiner

Ohio	20/40	20/30	20/70	20/60	Yes	—
Oklahoma	20/40	20/30	20/40	20/30	Yes	140°
Oregon	20/40	20/40	20/40	20/40	Yes	100°
Pennsylvania	20/40	20/40	20/40	20/40	Special cases	Special cases
Rhode Island	20/40	20/40	20/40	20/40	Yes	Standard practice
South Carolina	20/40	20/20	20/40	20/40	No	—
South Dakota	20/40	20/40	20/40	20/40	Yes	—
Tennessee	20/70	20/40	20/70	20/40	No	—
Texas	20/40	20/25	20/70	20/70	No	—
Utah	20/40	20/40	20/40	20/40	No	—
Vermont	20/40	20/40	20/40	20/40	Yes	100°
Virginia	20/40	20/40	20/40	20/40	No	100°
Washington	20/40	20/40	20/40	20/40	Fusion test replaces depth perception	—
West Virginia	20/40	20/40	20/40	20/40	Yes	—
Wisconsin	20/40	20/40	20/40	20/40	Yes	—
Wyoming	20/40	20/40	20/40	20/40	Yes	—

here are not always rigidly applied to each individual case. And if the applicant disagrees with the findings of his examiner, he has the right, in many cases, to have the results reviewed by a vision specialist.

The American Association of Motor Vehicle Administrators and the American Optometric Association, in a jointly published booklet on visual screening for driver licensing, remark that "Most drivers are anxious to retain driving privileges and as a result they learn to compensate for deficiencies."

Referring specifically to the one-eyed driver, the booklet states: "Since there is greatly impaired space perception, the person usually learns to utilize other cues such as shadows and perspective. One-eyed drivers learn or should be instructed to turn their heads from side to side frequently, especially if the right eye is the blind one. The reason for this seems to be that there may be more unobserved hazards approaching from the right side. A further safeguard for the one-eyed driver is the use of outside rearview mirrors."

I have yet to discover statistics on the safety record of one-eyed drivers. But most authorities I've talked to think their accident rate is no higher than that of persons with normal vision. Why should this be so? Because, say most of these experts, the one-eyed driver stays more alert.

PILOT LICENSING STANDARDS

The United States is one of several nations that takes an enlightened attitude about one-eyed fliers. Along with Canada and Australia, the U.S. will license one-eyed persons not only as private flyers but also as commercial pilots if they comply with certain procedures.

It was not always so. For many years candidate pilots were rejected for failure to pass the Howard Dolman depth perception test. This test required the person being tested to bring two vertical rods of identical size to approximately the same distance from the subject. This test does indeed screen out persons who do not have excellent binocular vision.

Eventually, however, aviation medical examiners began to question the relationship of the test to visual tasks involved in flying a plane. This liberalized position was taken only after years of research, testing and experimentation, culminating in some unusual landing tests. In this carefully controlled experiment, pilots with normal vision were asked to make a series of landings. After their performances were meticulously recorded, they were told to repeat the landings with one eye covered. *Their performance scores were identical*—even though the pilots complained that the one-eyed landings were more difficult. And considering that they were completely unadapted to monocular vision, that's hardly surprising.

Since landing a plane demands the most critical visual judgments of any flying task, earlier irrelevant tests were discarded and the rules relaxed for one-eyed fliers.

Today, when a licensed pilot loses the use of one eye, he is allowed an adaptation period of one year, during which he may fly with a student certificate. At the end of this period, a Federal Aviation Administration inspector tests him in such visual tasks as scanning the sky for traffic. When he passes this examination, he returns to normal flying status.

The success of this liberalized policy is attested by an F.A.A. study of air accidents made in 1965, which showed virtually no difference in the accident rate for one-eyed pilots from that of the total pilot population.

Even more important than that, however, is the singular *fact that no aviation accident has even been attributed to one-eyed vision!*

16

GREAT COMPANY

Throughout history people with all kinds of handicaps have distinguished themselves in all walks of life. Yet to the person who's facing the future with a newly acquired handicap, it's sometimes encouraging to take a look at some of the great company he'll find himself in. So just to end this book on an upbeat, let's call out a handful of the one-eyed greats—each of whom lost an eye comparatively late in life, yet never lost any momentum in living.

> A great British naval hero: Horatio Nelson.
> A great French Impressionist painter: Hilaire Germain Edgar Degas.
> A great American war correspondent: Floyd Phillips Gibbons.
> A great Israeli general: Moshe Dayan.
> A great American aviator: Wiley Post.
> A great American scientist, Nobel Prize winner: Dr. Julius Axelrod.
> A great American entertainer: Sammy Davis, Jr.

Nelson even used his blind eye to advantage in

the historic Battle of Copenhagen in 1801. His superior, Sir Hyde Parker, had signaled him to halt his attack on a Danish ship against what Parker considered very dubious odds. Nelson placed a telescope against his blind eye and, after a careful "look," told his aide, "I do not see the signal." He then proceeded with the attack, which was soon to become a part of Britain's proud naval history. Thus Nelson used his handicap to turn a potential defeat into a resounding victory.

Go thou and do likewise.